YOU CAN'T TAKE IT WITH YOU

'Memories are the greatest gift I can leave behind'

When Jane Tomlinson, a devoted mother of three, was told she had only months to live, she had to find a way to make the most of every moment. Supported by her husband Mike, she began to run – and the London Marathon was just a start. In 2004 Jane and her brother Luke undertook the Rome to Home cycle ride, with a papal blessing in the pannier of their tandem. Since then she has completed the legendary Florida Full Ironman Triathlon, and a gruelling cycle ride from San Francisco to New York, raising £1.4 million for cancer charities.

YOU CAN'T TAKE IT WITH YOU

YOU CAN'T TAKE IT WITH YOU

by

Jane & Mike Tomlinson

Magna Large Print Books
Long Preston, North Yorkshire,
BD23 4ND, England.

TOM

British Library Cataloguing in Publication Data.

Tomlinson, Jane & Mike
  You can't take it with you.

  A catalogue record of this book is
  available from the British Library

  ISBN   978-0-7505-2685-2

First published in Great Britain in 2006 by Simon & Schuster Ltd.

Copyright © 2006 by Laneheath Limited

Cover illustration © Johnny Ring by arrangement with
Simon & Schuster Ltd.

The right of Jane and Mike Tomlinson to be identified as the author of
this work has been asserted in accordance with sections 77 and 78 of
the Copyright, Designs and Patents Act, 1988

Published in Large Print 2007 by arrangement with
Simon & Schuster Ltd.

Magna Large Print is an imprint of Library Magna Books Ltd.

Printed and bound in Great Britain by
T.J. (International) Ltd., Cornwall, PL28 8RW

Picture Credits

To Suzanne, Rebecca and Steven
Still glad to be sharing time with you
Love, Mum and Dad

JANE

The white halogen light on the front of my bike bit into the gathering dark, illuminating just a few feet in front of me. The roads were lit by street lamps, yellow halos against the gathering gloom. The day had begun brightly, the sun refracting from the frost on the roadside in a myriad of shafts. Now that the sun had lowered, the cold made my thighs sting and my feet numb. My hands, covered with only a thin pair of running gloves, inadequate against the icy wind, were frozen. My shower-proof jacket flapped about my body, billowing coldness against my torso. The warm bright pub and roast beef dinner that my brother Luke and I had enjoyed hours earlier were long since forgotten and many miles away. We were still far from home.

We topped the small hill and I gladly slung low over the handlebars, raising my tender buttocks from the saddle and making the most of the effortless downhill. I pushed myself lower, streamlining my body in an effort to catch up with Luke ahead.

Three young lads stepped into the road, shouting at us as we screeched by. I heard snatched sounds but with the wind roaring in my ears, I was unable to make out their words. The road levelled out and ignoring the dullness in my legs, I pushed down and round on the pedals, hauling my feet up as I continued to chase Luke.

He slowed and I finally pedalled level with him. Away from the centre of Fairburn village the darkness closed in on all sides. The catseyes blinked at us, reflecting the dim beams of our lights as we rode past them.

'Did you hear what those lads shouted?' Luke asked.

'No, I thought they were just taking the piss,' I replied.

'They said we won't get through on this road. It must be flooded.'

'Oh great, the final turn-off was at the top of the last descent.'

I turned and looked over my shoulder at the road disappearing into an inky blackness. I was too tired to contemplate returning up the steep climb behind us. Luke looked at me, my shoulders slumped, my head dropping forwards through exhaustion.

'Let's just keep going,' he said. 'It can't be that bad.'

The silence on the unlit stretch of road was eerie as we pedalled side by side, the quietness broken by the marshy water lapping against the roadside. As we rounded a bend we could make out two red lights suspended above the road. Drawing closer we could see they belonged to the rear of a car, the two shafts of its headlights reflecting on the black still water ahead of us. The road, unseen below the water, stretched into the distance. We stopped and steadied the bikes. I looked from the flooded road to Luke.

'It'll be fine,' he said. I shook my head in disbelief. 'I'll go first and see how it is.'

I watched as Luke pushed down and set off cycling into the small black lake ahead. His bicycle wheels gradually submerged before disappearing below the water, forcing him to dismount the bike. I could still make out the red light on the rear of his bike glowing from beneath the water, then appearing again as Luke passed through the deepest part and made his way out of the flood. He turned and yelled back at me. 'Come on. It's not that bad, just take it slowly.'

I sat up on the saddle of the bike and pushed on the pedals, cycling nervously into the water. The dark eddies swirled as the wheels cut through the black lake. The bike lurched, deep water braking my progress. I climbed off, lowering my feet on to the unseen ground, and pushed forward. The water crept over my knees, up my thighs and then it was just below my waist. Wading slowly, I gasped as the chill lapped against me and con-strained my breath. As I neared Luke at the other side, relief made me rush forward.

Luke, shaking with the cold, bent to empty water from his shoes. I looked at him and became aware that my own feet – no longer numbed by the frozen water – ached, chilled with pain. I sat on the wet tarmac, my lower body no longer bothered by the water, and tried to force my fingers to fumble the knot of my trainer open. 'I can't untie this,' I said, my eyes screwing up, my voice coming out as a childish whine, fed up now with the cold.

I was hungry, tired and in the middle of nowhere. The morning had been icily beautiful when I had phoned Luke to ask if he wanted to go for a bike ride. We had set our sights on a round trip to Selby and back. It would mean a fifty-mile round-trip, further than either of us had ventured before. However, we had set out too late, and lingered too long over a rich pub lunch. We should have turned back then, but looking at the map over lunch I spotted the small town of Cawood.

'What do you reckon?' I had asked, tracing the route. 'Or we could head back now.'

Our eyes searched the map – it didn't look too far. It was a decision I had started to regret as we wheeled the bikes over the bridge spanning the motorway at Fairburn. The street lamps were just starting to come on at the end of the day. Mike hadn't sounded too happy when I spoke to him on the phone.

'Do you want me to come out and meet you?' he asked. I was too headstrong – too independent – to acknowledge that I might need my husband's help.

The knot still wouldn't budge and Luke knelt down and worked it loose. Pulling my trainer off he emptied out the water. He took my socks and walked away from me.

'What are you doing?' I asked, laughing, as I watched him wringing my sodden socks out into the lake in the road.

'What?'

'As if it matters if you get water on the road!' I giggled. Luke began to laugh too.

It was another fifty minutes before we were pushing the pedals along the stretch of road towards Rothwell. There was no pretence now at trying to keep up with Luke. Setting my face against the aches and pains that seemed to be in every part of me, I just wanted to get off the saddle. I tugged again at my damp trousers trying to stop them rubbing the soft part of my thighs.

On the last little hill to our estate and even in the lowest gear it felt like I was pushing too hard and that the bike would come to a halt beneath me. I kept my legs moving round, using sheer willpower to get me home.

The light was on outside the house and I propped the bike against the wall. Leaving my trainers outside, I opened the door and collapsed on to the stairs to ease my sodden leggings from my bluey white legs. Wrapping a towel around my waist I threw a warm towel at Luke, who was similarly disrobing.

Half-dressed and enjoying the warmth of the fire in the living room, my hands were clenched around a steaming mug of coffee. Mike sat opposite Luke and me, his face set, his eyes narrowed, his hands clenched in his lap from hours of anxiety turned to fury.

'That wasn't very grown-up was it?' he said quietly. Luke and I sat like two schoolchildren being admonished by a teacher.

'I'm sorry,' I muttered. 'It was too cold and too late to look for another phone box, we thought we'd better just get back.'

'It isn't just that,' Mike said. 'I was worried that you weren't lit up well enough to be out on the roads this late.'

I watched Mike through the steam from my drink as he continued frowning at me. Luke and I knew our mistake but we were hardly likely to admit it to Mike. He rose from the settee and left the room, shrugging his shoulders in disgust. Luke and I looked at each other hardly daring to smile.

'Dad's a bit grumpy isn't he?' Luke whispered.

CHAPTER 1

January 2003

MIKE

Suzanne curled her legs beneath her torso, taking a lengthy gulp from her drink.

'Suzanne!' Rebecca laughed.

'What?' Suzanne feigned surprise.

'Glug, glug, glug – it's like someone emptying a drain.'

Suzanne's face turned to a sulk but unable to keep up the pretence she cracked a smile. I looked at the three of them sharing a sofa. Jane and Rebecca were concentrating on *ER* while Suzanne, who didn't share their love of medical dramas, was shrieking at every bloodthirsty moment and being a bit of a girl about the whole thing. Strange how she found it more palatable than revising for her A levels.

It had never really occurred to me how much the two girls looked like their mum. But looking at them, with their slim physiques, blue eyes and same-shaped faces, the similarities were obvious. While strangers had often said to me how alike they were, I never usually saw it.

'Who'd like a fresh coffee and ice cream?' Jane asked. The girls nodded enthusiastically. 'Go on Mike,' she said.

I wasn't keen to leave the cosy heat of the living room for the five-yard walk outside into the lashing sleet to the freezer in the garage, so I did my best to ignore her.

'Go on, go on, go on, go on,' she pleaded, pulling a sad face with cow eyes. She was soon joined by the other two. It was pointless to resist. I walked through the hall where a rustle on the stairs attracted my attention. I looked up and saw Steven, motionless at the top step, his legs on the step below, his elbows resting on his knees, hand cupping his chin.

'What's up?' I asked.

'I can't get to sleep.'

'Have you tried?'

'I had a bad dream.'

'I thought you couldn't get to sleep.'

'I was asleep, but can't now because I had a bad dream.'

'What was it about?'

'Can't remember.'

His cheeks widened to a smile that would have thawed an iceberg. Squinting my eyes to show a serious fatherly face, I said, 'Bed.'

'Okay.'

Minutes later with ice creams and coffee loaded on a tray, I returned to the living room. To my surprise Steven was perched on his mum's knee. They both shot me a conspiratorial smile and I noticed Steven's eyes glinting – he knew full well he had put one over on me.

Handing out the coffees, I retook my seat and looked across to the four of them. It seemed that so much time had passed and so much had happened since that dreadful day in Settle two and half years ago when Jane and I had to break the news that she was dying. Seated in my parents' living room, Jane had explained why the tickly cough, breathlessness, loss of balance and bone pains were symptoms of spreading breast cancer that, according to the consultant, would take Jane's life in six months.

Now I'd occasionally forget Jane was ill. To me, she was seemingly indestructible, all those marathons, triathlons and awards. How could she have something inside her that was slowly killing her? But those illusions were shattered too often and too quickly when bouts of illness or scans would reaffirm the disease's progressive nature. There was a question I'd asked myself then and asked myself over and over in the months following Jane's diagnosis – but how could I be their mum?

If it was a difficult situation to get my head round in August 2000, now, in January 2003, it was impossible. Jane's ability to continue functioning normally as mother, wife, domestic slave, radiographer and fundraiser gave her an aura of invincibility. I couldn't compare.

Suzanne was due to go to university in September and the dynamics of the family would inevitably change. But that was planned; it would be temporary and, more importantly, out of choice. Jane's inevitable absence on the other hand... A sadness overwhelmed me, and my chest heaved tightly.

'Mike, are you all right?' Jane asked.

'Yes, why wouldn't I be?' I said with a marked lack of joy.

It had not occurred to me that Jane would still be alive when Suzanne went to university. Not long after being told Jane had only six months to live, I had mentally totted up what ages Rebecca and Steven would be when their older sister left the nest and how it would affect Rebecca being the oldest female at home.

'Mike! Mike!'

I looked at Jane and realised four pairs of eyes were staring at me. 'Are you with us? Tuck Steven in; it's the adverts and cheer up, you miserable git.'

After taking Steven to his bed I sat on the top step listening to the sounds echoing through the house, the hum of the fridge, the radio from Rebecca's empty room, laughter from the living room. Normal. Too normal.

Jane, as always, seemed imperturbable. Even the new Vinorelbine chemotherapy, which she had been undergoing for eight weeks, had barely altered her daily life. Ever the optimist, she always felt glad for what she had. Meanwhile, I just felt sorry for what I'd lose. I couldn't live like this.

'Dad, I can see you.' Steven was curled near the foot of his bed.

'Goodnight, Steven, get back into bed.'

'Mike, what are you doing?' Jane shouted.

There was no sanctuary, no solitude at home. Thank goodness.

A few days later Jane and I found ourselves alighting from a train at Stalybridge station nestled in the Pennines. A sharp January wind took away our breath and as the train continued on its way to Manchester it left the platform bereft of any life except us. Now our ears were no longer ringing to the optimistic chants of football fans going to the match, our surroundings seemed like cold-war Berlin. Bracing ourselves to battle against the flying paper missiles caused by the platform's wind-tunnel effect, we headed to the station café.

Entering was like walking into a time capsule and into a 1950s-style scene, the type you would find on a cosy Sunday evening family drama. A tall, well-built man walked towards us and in a rich Mancunian accent said, 'Mike, Jane, can I get you a beer?' We shook hands.

'Good to see you, Craig,' I said. Craig is an old friend who I'd met when we studied law together at Manchester Polytechnic and he now doubled as our solicitor.

Jane moved to give him a hug. Stalybridge's station café seemed to have been immune from the franchised characterless counterparts in bigger stations. It served proper food and, more importantly, real ale. My stomach was reminding me that it had just gone twelve. 'Have you eaten, Craig?'

'We had something before we came out.'

'I'll have a growler and a pint.' Jane had gone to join Craig's fiancée, Ann, at the table. 'You'd better get a pint for Jane as well, Craig.'

Halfway through the first pint, Craig leant

down to retrieve a leather folder not dissimilar to something you would expect a Second World War spy to carry. He brought out some legal documents. 'You had better get these signed before you get too pissed to do them.'

There was something rather sobering about the stiff parchment and old-fashioned font that read 'Last Will and Testament'.

'Has she left everything to me, Craig?' I asked.

'Not that you deserve it...' he said.

'In that case let her sign it.'

Jane, who had been peering down at the document, raised a quizzical eye.

'It is one of the downsides of living so long, the extra expense of an updated will,' I quipped.

Jane shot me a look. I beamed a smile and said, 'Only joking, you know I love you.'

'No you don't. I'm just a cash cow for you so you can be wealthy after I'm gone.' The frown held for thirty seconds before she smiled.

The catalyst for making the will had been Jane's imminent adventure. It's a reminder of mortality that few relish but with Jane there was the added knowledge that these instructions would need to be carried out in the not-too-distant future.

Craig's only fee for his fine legal services was that we accompanied him and Ann on a twelve-hour bender. We duly obliged. When our senses were completely dulled we headed for a curry; is there a better way of sealing your last testament?

Although the idea to cycle from John o'Groats to Land's End to raise money for charity had germinated the previous summer, it was only now in the first month of 2003 that we could begin to plan with any certainty. Jane's illness and the realisation that her health could change in a matter of weeks rather than months meant that all our efforts had to be concertinaed into a short space of time.

Because of this tight timeline, the opportunity to fundraise was limited. It also meant that planning was difficult. Without the advantages of a pool of money to fund equipment we knew we were in need of support if the bike ride was to go ahead. News presenter Harry Gration at the BBC in Leeds had advised us to contact Len McCormick and Ian Dyson of Batleys Plc, whom he said had fine charitable instincts and were inspired by Jane's efforts in the previous year.

Three days after our meeting with Craig and with a hangover still lingering, Jane and I sat in the car park at Batleys' head office waiting to put forward our proposition.

'What are you going to say, Mike?'

I looked at Jane in the passenger seat noticing her eyelids half-closed, her shoes barely protecting her feet from the damp and miserable day.

'I'm just going to wing it,' I said. 'Either they'll want to help or they won't.'

I smiled, hoping to reassure Jane, but her gaze focused into the distance. I had funded last year's events out of our own family budget but we were both aware that we couldn't afford to do that again this year.

I'd underestimated how difficult it would be to get assistance for the cycle ride, even with Jane winning awards and her media exposure. While a lot of people gave platitudes and pats on the back, so far we'd had no financial assistance.

We were met by the impressive form of Ian Dyson, the marketing director, and Len McCormick. Both had vice-like handshakes and a direct manner. Batleys had sponsored the BBC Yorkshire and Lincolnshire Sports Awards in December where Jane had won the Special Award, so Len had met Jane previously.

'Come in, come in. It is good to see you, Jane, how are you?' Len's scouse accent and warm pleasant manner immediately made us feel at home. 'Well, what are you planning and how do you think we can help you?'

'We are setting up an appeal to help a number of charities for children as well as cancer charities. While cancer affects Jane's life it doesn't define her. She works with children who are in a much less fortunate position than ourselves. Neither of us know how we'd cope if this illness was happening to one of the kids rather than Jane.'

Len nodded. His mind seemed to move quickly. 'And you are setting off from Scotland?' Len asked. 'Why that way round – don't most people go from Land's End to John o'Groats?'

'We'd prefer to take the harder route,' shrugged Jane, 'and we are hoping to get more publicity later in the ride where the population's denser. That way we'll raise more money. Hopefully a hundred thousand pounds.'

Finally, Len cracked a smile. 'How about if we cover the food and accommodation? But don't skimp. Make sure Jane's comfortable, and Ian

23

will give you a hand with the marketing, too, if you'd like.'

Jane and I smiled our thanks.

By the time we left the building, daylight had disappeared. 'So, what did you think?' Jane asked as we walked back to the car.

'It's a result, but they have brought up a load of questions about how I will raise the money, how underprepared we are and how risky it is for you. You're not well, you have got no bike equipment and you will be up in Scotland on your own. You will need chemo and we will need to bring you back every week. I am not sure how we can manage to do this.'

'It will be all right Mike,' said Jane.

'Shouldn't it be me saying that?'

JANE

The prospect of the cycle ride had given my confidence a huge boost. All winter I had put off climbing on to the bike fearing that my frequent bouts of light-headedness would make cycling too difficult. I was still undergoing chemotherapy but I wasn't sure it was doing any good. Every week I went to the hospital to have concoctions dripped into me. Every Friday I had the same tiredness, limbs heavy, aching as though I was just starting with the flu. My stomach felt full and acid reared up my throat, accompanied by nausea.

The feelings of clumsiness, of the world lurching away from me, still hadn't receded and the pain in my shoulder and my leg made sleep difficult. Struggling home to fall into bed drop-dead tired, I was unable to face any domestic chores until I had rested.

I had promised Rebecca the summer before that I would find a triathlon for her to take part in that year. She fancied the swimming, cycling and running and wanted to see what it was like so I bought the January edition of *220 Triathlon* magazine hoping to find an event for her in the diary section. Flicking through the magazine on the bus journey home, I looked at the dates but could see nothing suitable for Rebecca. I turned to the front page and read through the editor's words describing the inaugural half ironman at Sherborne in Dorset later that year. The half ironman was an incredibly tough event, not something I could ever contemplate; my feeble body wouldn't manage a whole day's physical exertion. Still I was intrigued enough to read the article outlining the course. It looked a fabulous setting; the swim was in the lake set in the castle grounds. The ride out into Dorset countryside passed the chalk drawing of the white naked man in the hills above. The run looked beautiful but tough – mixed terrain through woods, across fields and down farm-tracks. The distances seemed incomprehensible – the swim 1900 metres in open water, the bike ride a-not-too-hilly fifty-six miles, as well as a half marathon.

Still the idea appealed to me. But fifty-six miles on a bike? Luke and I had barely managed that the previous weekend. My buttocks still ached, my back was stiff and I had been unwilling to let Mike know how much my legs had suffered. I didn't want to allow him to declare with that smug look on his face that I should have been more sensible. There was no way I could cycle fifty-six miles and then run a half marathon but part of me felt swayed by the notion.

'I'll just start tea then,' I said to Mike later that evening. I sat at the kitchen table peeling potatoes, the sharp knife sliding under the pale brown skin. I knew my limitations. Peeling spuds was one task I could manage; dicing vegetables was a whole different story with my present lack of coordination.

Mike sat opposite me and picked up the triathlon magazine.

'I thought I might find a triathlon for Rebecca but the half ironman triathlon looks stunning. It would be an awesome event to be part of, but my body just wouldn't be able to cope.'

'Why don't you think about it?' Mike said. 'After all you'll have the perfect training, cycling from John o'Groats to Land's End. That should get you fit enough.'

I turned towards him and raised my eyebrows. 'I'll think about it,' I said.

MIKE

Completing the Brass Monkey Half Marathon at York had been the acid test to see whether Jane would be able to even contemplate doing the cycle ride. She'd passed it triumphantly, so the adventure could begin. But with only six weeks to go, we needed to think about sharing plans with the media.

From the previous year's experiences with the marathon, we knew there were three key moments when we could optimise awareness of the event and therefore raise the most money – announcing the adventure, the few days just before they set off and the few days after they'd finished.

Because of Jane's precarious health we were reluctant to announce plans too early, though we realised that restricted the amount of unsolicited support that would come to us. With Jane's fitness improved and knowing that she could handle the chemotherapy, it was time to go public.

Jane sat in the living room as a stream of journalists asked about the trip, while I sat in the kitchen coordinating and making endless cups of tea. Rather than conduct a press conference – which to me seems a bit egotistical – we had contacted some people in the local media whom we'd dealt with over the last six months and asked if they would be interested in interviewing Jane. I was surprised by the take-up of invitations and I cleared a day out of our diary and arranged various appointments throughout the day. By eleven that morning, a collection of twenty used mugs was testament to the number of media people who had traipsed through the hall to the living room.

The door to the kitchen opened. 'Bye Mike,' said a voice. It was Chris Kiddy, the Yorkshire Television reporter, who poked his head round the door and waved. Meanwhile, Lia, a petite young blonde girl wearing boots and a belted overcoat, was trying to stand as unobtrusively as possible in our cramped kitchen.

'Hello Jane, I'm Lia.' Jane looked nonplussed at another stranger clutching a steaming mug. Lia continued, 'From the Press Association.'

Jane looked across at me, the dark marks under her eyes and sunken cheeks were not just as a result of the strain of today. 'I'm just going to take five minutes,' she barked quite abruptly, grabbing the door handle and vanishing.

I gave Lia an apologetic shrug and she smiled. We'd never really dealt with the Press Association before – it seemed rather grand. Lia, whom we'd never met, had sent us a Christmas card. Opening it, a business card floated to the floor. A lovely handwritten note invited us to contact her if we needed any help in the future. We'd recently called her – and after an inordinate number of delays and confusion she'd arrived.

Next to her I felt positively ancient. I felt like asking her if she was playing truant. After five minutes, Jane returned to the kitchen, interrupting Lia whose conversation was in full flow. At which point I heard an enthusiastic knock at the front door. 'I'll get it,' I shouted through to Jane.

'Ian Dovaston, *Sky News*. This is Martyn, my cameraman,' said a tall, dark-haired, skinny man with a Wearside accent. Well groomed and smartly dressed in a suit, he was immediately affable. Martyn, partially obscured by Ian, was similarly lean and tall with glasses and was poking his head round like a cheeky schoolboy. I showed them both in, leading them to the living room.

'Hi, Jane. Ian Dovaston, *Sky News*,' said Ian, spotting Jane in the kitchen. He sounded like he was signing off one of his news reports. Jane

28

looked at Ian, then at Lia, then at me.

'It's okay, Jane, speak to them first,' Lia said. 'I'll only have to go back to Hull and stand outside in the cold.'

'We won't be long,' Jane said firmly.

I watched as Martyn set up his equipment, camera and lighting gear in the living room while Ian checked out the Sports Personality trophy on the mantelpiece. Jane positioned herself in the camera's eye in anticipation of Martyn's next request. Sensing that I was redundant, I left to rejoin Lia, closing the doors to allow the sound recording not to be spoilt. I'd predicted the interview would take a maximum of five minutes but after thirty I thought I should check on progress and ensure Jane was okay. I found them all, off camera, totally engrossed in conversation about the ride's details, logistics and planning.

Martyn, who was unplugging the audio cables, looked at me. 'I've been telling Jane that I've always wanted to cycle the end to end. It'll be fantastic, a life's experience, I'm so jealous.' His enthusiasm was infectious. Laughing, he kept saying, 'I can't believe you're doing this.'

Ian said, 'Me too; what a journey.' Martyn was still chuckling as he wandered down the drive back to the car.

Three days later, Ian called asking if he and Martyn could join Jane on the ride.

JANE

I sat in the treatment room, in the oncology out-

29

patients at St James's University Hospital, along with ten other patients. Some faces were familiar, others were new to me.

I watched as Catherine, the nurse, prepared the sterile trolley, going through the same routine I'd witnessed so often before. Pulling open the metal drawer which screeched metal against metal, she removed the files and syringes, readying herself.

Mentally detached from this part of the procedure I sat day-dreaming as she attached a syringe of saline to the end of the special canula – the tube – that would be inserted into my portocath that was positioned in my upper arm.

Thanks to my medical background, I knew a little about the different types of catheters that could be used and had been positive that the portocath was the best option for me. Not only would it allow me to run and to swim but it also meant I could work as normal in the radiography department. Other catheters could have spread infection and I would have been banned from performing certain duties, but with a portocath there was no danger. It is a closed system which gives doctors access to a line in the top of my arm which is clean and sterile. When the needle is removed from the skin there is no opening that could lead to an infection. I'd asked for it after having only a couple of chemo sessions. The chemotherapy caused some nausea and tiredness but I also got muscular spasm and pain in the area that it was injected into, which took up to five days to calm. The weekly injections meant that there were very few pain-free days and the redness and swelling were alarming. The portocath meant that the chemotherapy went straight into a large vein, so I would not get the swelling and pain.

Initially the medical team were reluctant to give into my wishes – after all, it's one of the more expensive options – but after stating my case on several occasions to both the nursing staff and my consultant, they capitulated.

I shuddered as Catherine held up a monstrously long needle tapered at the end. She knelt and placed the fingers of her left hand to steady the nipple of the catheter and then plunged the needle straight in. My leg straightened unconsciously and my back muscles tightened, my feet arched. My face screwed up as Catherine attached an empty syringe and pulled back on the plunger. The plunger was reluctant to move and Catherine put her head to one side, 'Sorry.' Pulling back on the syringe again, this time dark-red blood flowed in so she clicked the line shut and attached a second empty syringe to siphon off more blood. She hung a bag of saline from the drip stand and labelled the phials of my blood ready to send them to the lab to check my blood counts and make sure my body was robust enough to cope with another session of chemotherapy.

My blood counts had been dropping since the start of my chemo. The normal haemoglobin levels of thirteen were down to below ten. I was tired and, though I wasn't breathless, the stairs seemed increasingly steep as I crept up them. In fact I'd taken to avoiding climbing them and making the journey up to the bedrooms only when really necessary. A blood transfusion before

Christmas had helped, but then my levels had started to fall once more.

The last review appointment with Dr Perrin had been fairly routine. Scans of my head had not shown any reason for my loss of balance. It was possible that the low blood levels were contributing to it.

'We could put you on EPO,' Dr Perrin had suggested. 'It will boost the bone marrow and make your body produce more red blood cells. It's pretty unusual to use it for the Vinorelbine regime,' he continued, 'but there is a precedent set in that we use it for the younger testicular cancer patients. I think with the level of activity you're involved in we could argue for its necessity to maintain your quality of life.'

I was always glad when we had these kind of discussions with Dr Perrin. Unlike some oncologists, he had an open mind as to how I could be treated in line with what I wanted to achieve in my life. I very much felt that he was treating me and not my disease. Without addressing the drop in my haemoglobin levels, how could I possibly anticipate the bicycle ride Mike and I were still tentatively planning? The recent York half marathon had been a hard physical challenge, but I had made it round and here I was contemplating a cycle ride of over 1000 miles.

My chemotherapy couldn't be postponed. I would just have to find some way of getting back from the bike ride to Leeds for the weekly treatment. My chemo always fell on a Wednesday and, if I could, I usually used it as a rest day. The chemotherapy made me feel nauseous and, although it was never enough to actually vomit, my nose would wrinkle at strong smells and my stomach would lurch when my senses told me something unpleasant was in the air. The Herceptin made me feel like my throat and nose were swollen with a cold coming on. My limbs felt achy and heavy and I would head straight to bed when I finally arrived home.

On other days I managed to fit in some training. I would climb on to the saddle of the static bike at the gym, letting my legs go round and round while listening to the same twelve songs on my mini-disc player. There was a pleasing monotony to it. Increasing the time I spent on the bike each occasion I went, it was only a matter of weeks before I was cycling for ninety minutes at a time. Splitting up the time in my head into ten-minute mental hurdles, I would simply concentrate on the music and on turning and turning my legs.

Luke and I had been out training on the roads too. One cold day in March, we cycled down the same stretch of road we'd been down just a couple of months before. This time, instead of frost, the weather was wet and windy. But each time I thought I'd had just about enough of my wet trousers chaffing my thighs, the sun would appear and my clothing would dry out just enough to be bearable until the next downpour. My legs felt strong and I was enjoying myself until Luke set off up one steep climb just past Lotherton Hall, about ten miles into our ride.

I dropped down to the smallest ring and down through the gears until I had slowed so much that I could only decrease my pace further if I jumped off and pushed the damn thing up the hill. A squeaking and creaking from just behind nearly made me lose my concentration. The battered blue frame of an ancient road bike gradually crept past me. Its owner was a woman in a blue anorak. Her hood was pulled up over her head to keep off the rain but, even so, it didn't hide the fact that she was clearly of advancing years. Struggling to match her pace, I had plenty of time to watch as she squinted at me from behind her metal-framed spectacles and drew ahead of me. As she overtook with some ease, I could see her bicycle rack with a few groceries in it. The indignity of it made me dig deep and I really pushed down to try to keep her from cresting the hill before me.

Despite my efforts she was long gone before I got there. Luke also had plenty of time to sit at the top of the hill and observe my exertions. 'Well, at least you didn't get off and walk,' he said wryly. Pink-faced and shamed I offered no reply, worried about the distances we would soon be travelling and the inclines we were likely to meet.

'What else have you got planned this week?' asked Luke when we finally arrived back at my home.

'I thought I might go for a longish run.'

'You're not still thinking of running the marathon are you?' he asked. 'You're mad.'

Neither of us was sure how three weeks of cycling would affect our stamina or our running but as we both had places on the London Marathon for the weekend we hoped to finish the ride, I at least wanted to try to run the twenty-six miles at the end of our epic journey.

MIKE

My dad's deterioration since Christmas had shocked us all. Rebecca, who had spent most of her Christmas holidays with my parents up in Settle, had alluded to his confusion on her return but I had not paid sufficient attention to her anecdotes. She doted on her granddad but our concentration was elsewhere.

Dad had experienced spells of confusion before but his lucidity had always recovered to a large extent after each episode, although it seemed never to recover fully to the starting position. However, nothing had prepared me for when I first visited him in hospital in January. He hadn't recognised me and although I had tried to convince myself that there had been a hint of him knowing who I was, in my heart I knew I was merely deluding myself.

It seemed to me that we were watching someone becoming unfamiliar with the world. On each visit, another skill would have been lost. On Saturday mornings we visited as a family, on Tuesday or Wednesday I would either go alone or with Suzanne or Rebecca – sometimes both. With Jane setting off on Thursday morning I was desperate to get up once more midweek so I had squeezed in an extra Tuesday visit.

Driving up at six-thirty after work, it was already pitch black and it seemed inconceivable that Jane would be starting riding on Friday. The journey provided some respite from the breakneck pace of the last two weeks and time to consider that, while logistically the ride seemed to be going to plan, the fundraising efforts had begun to unravel.

A bizarre unsolicited phone call from the BBC last Friday asked if we were going to postpone the ride, as the war in Iraq would start on Monday. Quite how or why they would know such detail was a surprise, but the journalist was convinced. The call came just as other TV, radio and newspapers started cancelling interviews as various media organisations adjusted their schedules.

It took me a second to realise that, whatever anyone else's plans were, the ride would continue. Jane's health meant that we had no guarantees of her continued wellbeing. We had all worked so damned hard to get this far that we weren't going to be diverted. When we set up the ride we were aware that the inclement weather could cause problems and I knew the fundraising wouldn't be as successful this time, but at least Jane was on the start line.

Arriving at Airedale Hospital the weather was bleak and the likelihood that my dad would have further deteriorated saddened my heart. With my mind miles away, I fumbled with the two-handled door to the ward which provoked a tut from Rebecca. 'Well, if you can do better,' I retorted, which she promptly did.

Rebecca marched off purposefully down the straight fifty yards to the reception area, which was strategically placed to allow a good view of both main corridors. Security in the patients' interest was tight and not dissimilar to a well-run nursery.

Three years ago Belinda Archer, Jane's breast care nurse, told me on the night of Jane being diagnosed with incurable breast cancer not to have any hope. False hope would benefit no one. Human nature as it is would cling to any loosely worded sentences, seeing hope where there was none.

It was hard banishing any notion that Jane could be cured – either by medical breakthrough or a wrong diagnosis. In my head, I knew that the doctors were right and that she would die but in my heart I wanted to believe that their knowledge was not complete. And, of course, as Jane had lived, that desire to believe they were wrong had a stronger pull. But with each set of scans, that flicker of hope was extinguished only to reignite as time moved on.

It was a similar situation with Dad. Since his illness had been diagnosed I had grasped at the faintest glimpse of increased lucidity; spotting non-existent differences as a beacon for brighter days ahead. It was clear, though, that his decline was continuing and with each passing week his brain shut down further. Sometimes, on first seeing him, he was barely recognisable as the dad who had always been a larger-than-life figure for me. Watching my hero's faculties disappear was heartbreaking.

On entering the large common room, the UEFA theme song was vibrating the TV in preparation for the night's Champions' League match. I saw my dad and shook his right hand while I put my left on his shoulder. His frame was still solid although I had never seen him as light.

Rebecca rushed up to hug him, Suzanne was more circumspect.

'Hello, granddad,' she said. Of course, there was no response.

Some patients were seated around the room, others were walking in abstract directions. All were clean, dressed and comfortable.

While Rebecca fussed over my dad she gave a monologue of her day and how Jane was preparing for the trip. I was filled with an enormous sense of pride that she could hide her own hurt and show such tenderness. While she was busy, I spotted a blue balloon, partly obscured by a footstool, nestling under a chair. Once I had liberated it, Suzanne and I started passing it between us with our feet.

Suddenly, there was a glint in my dad's eyes as he joined in the game. It was the image of my childhood, his mischievous grin radiating the room. He had forgotten who we were, but was able to instinctively control the balloon and pass it back. For fifteen minutes we rolled back the years until the other patients' complaints became too loud and vociferous. Once finished, my dad's smile vanished and he disappeared from our world.

I felt uplifted on my arrival home knowing that my dad would be proud of Jane's efforts. Opening the front door, the alarm gave three sharp shrills to announce our return. 'Jane,' I yelled, partly to let her know it was us, partly to find out which room she was in. As our car is a diesel and sounds like a clapped-out tractor, rattling windows and bins as it makes its progress up the street, there is no real need to say, 'Only me', but we still do. There was no response so I went upstairs to the bedroom. Jane was sat propped up by a pillow, suitcases spread out in front of her, talking to herself. 'Are you all right?' I asked.

'Sshhh.'

'Are you losing it?'

'Shut up!'

Jane pointed to her camcorder on the bookshelf, which seemed self-defeating. Reluctantly she had agreed to my request to do a video diary for the BBC's local news. As a consequence every time she used it, it reminded her that it was my fault, so it was advisable for me to beat a retreat. 'Luke's collected the motorhome,' she said as I edged through the door.

'What's it like?'

'Four wheels, big and white, plastered with the appeal and company logos.'

'Yes, but what's it like?'

'It's a fucking motorhome, Michael. They all look the same, just this one's got the appeal logo on it.'

'How big is the lettering? Is there plenty of room? Is it easy to drive?'

'If you were that interested you'd have gone with Luke to pick it up. Now, go away!'

I shut the bedroom door, dodged the clothes-horse festooned with luminous cycling gear on the landing. The house was turning into a cycling warehouse; boxes of powdered Lucozade Sport, Mars bars and Glenfiddich were everywhere. I felt stung by Jane after I had helped organise the ride. It was childish but now I felt my face was being put out. The cycling siblings were a better team than Jane and I ever would have been. Luke was far more practical than me, a natural athlete too. As an A&E nurse, his medical knowledge would be invaluable whereas I couldn't even apply a plaster. Here he was at the end of a long stretch of nights but he had still summoned enough energy to collect the motorhome.

The motorhome had been the result of an unsolicited offer from a kind gentleman in Rotherham who ran a motorhome business. It had been a real godsend providing at once accommodation for a support team, a mobile café for the cyclists, a motorised billboard and a sense of professionalism to the outside world. It was to be manned by Jane's Uncle Richard, nicknamed Captain Dick as a recognition of his seafaring profession, and his son Chris, Jane's cousin. Two people whose scouse dialect was unfathomable to anyone who didn't listen carefully.

There was a mix of trepidation and excitement in the house, although as the hours passed I seemed further distanced from the hub. All day I had been speaking to people heading up to John o'Groats, the cyclists, support crew and media. I'd organised the party but wasn't going to be there. I was envious of Jane, not of the attention but of the adventure I'd miss. Also, as I was ultimately responsible for the finance and logistics of the ride, being hundreds of miles away was going to be difficult to take.

The transit-camp feel spread to the living room where an ordnance survey map was laid out over the coffee table. Both girls busied themselves with menial jobs, an effort not to draw their parents' attentions. Suzanne was only weeks away from her A levels and the house was full of distractions – visitors, the phone constantly ringing. Jane's departure should ease the pressure.

As evening drew to a close we curtailed our desperate activities to share a few moments' conversation, while the TV provided background noise. It wasn't long though before it became the focal point of our attentions as the pictures from Baghdad were showing the start of hostilities. The images became sickly compelling – slow-motion action replays of bombs hitting their targets. It reminded me of a night twelve years previously, shortly after Jane had been diagnosed with breast cancer, when similar pictures were being shown. I contemplated sadly how little some things change.

JANE

'Why isn't somebody answering the telephone?' I thought as a shrill intermittent beeping entered into my subconscious. I roused myself roughly from sleep as the sound became more urgent, getting louder and louder until it eventually filled the room and my head. I reached out from the bed and felt around on the tall bedside cabinet for the alarm clock. It thudded to the ground, continuing to shriek, louder and quicker. Cursing I untangled myself from the bed covers and crouched down to search for the clock in my clothes scattered at the side of the bed. Finally, I picked it up and pushed the switch to stop the noise.

Mike shuffled on the other side of the bed, burrowing himself into its warmth. 'I'll be up in a minute,' he muttered wearily.

I switched on the bedroom light, its glaring brightness making my tired eyes screw up. Still clutching my alarm clock, I pushed it into the depths of my suitcase, its contents groaning against even the smallest extra item. Everything I would be wearing for the next three weeks was in there. Cycle shoes, shorts, tops, jackets and waterproofs, dayglo green. There was barely room left for any non-biking clothes, but I couldn't sleep without my pyjamas, and I had some essential reading books. I felt lost without some reading matter. Alongside all the clothes and books was my itinerary – the route, maps and hotel bookings for the journey from John o'Groats to Land's End. I pushed hard on to the top of the case and forced the zip round. I tried lifting it, but found the strain too much and left it where it was.

I moved as quietly as I could down the stairs and knocked on the living-room door, easing it open. I could make out the worm-like figure of my brother Luke in his sleeping bag. He groaned, shaking his head slightly as if to throw off the tiredness.

'I'm up,' he mumbled, as he unzipped his bag.

I closed the door and made my way into the kitchen, filling the kettle and turning it on for a much needed coffee. It was just after 4.30 a.m. The early start was necessary to allow us to drive all the way up to the northernmost tip of Scotland so we could arrive there late afternoon and be ready to start cycling our epic journey the next day. The kitchen door squeaked and Luke's face appeared, lined and heavy with tiredness. He'd had only four hours' sleep in the last twenty-four and he had just finished his night shifts the day before.

My sleep had been light, starting awake as I tried to go through all the lists of essential equipment. The small whisky I'd had before bedtime had made me sleepy but had not kept me asleep. My nerves and fears over what lay ahead raced through my mind. The hard days cycling, the media schedules and intrusions. Would everyone be rooting for me, or were they going to follow me on my journey to watch me fail?

I longed to have only the naive worries of childhood that I remembered seeing in Suzanne as a small girl. I pictured her hair and open sunny face.

Suzanne tugged at my hand and I looked down at her clad in her blue teddy sweater knitted by her grandma, her ragged fringe framing her face held up towards me. 'Mummy!'

'What's the matter?' Her big blue eyes were heavy with unfallen tears. Her teeth chewed at her full bottom lip, her chin dimpled and creased with the effort of not crying. I knelt down. 'What is it?' I asked.

'I put a penny in and it won't let me have an egg.' She pointed to the large curved cage with a gaudy coloured parrot in it.

'What penny?' I asked, shuffling forwards in the queue.

'My penny from my penny box.' She couldn't con-

43

tain herself any longer, and the tears rolled down her face. 'I put my penny in. It was mine, Mummy, but I didn't get an egg.' She was talking quickly, gulping down the sobs.

I handed my signed child allowance book over the counter and waited as my meagre monies were passed over, shoving the pounds in my bag. Just then my stomach lurched as the baby inside me elbowed or kicked against my taut belly. I clutched Suzanne's hand feeling the warmth as she clung to me. We made our way to the toy machine. I turned the handle and Suzanne's brown much-fingered two-pence piece fell out. 'Is this it?'

'Yes. It's my penny.'

'I think you need a silver penny for this.' I handed her a twenty-pence piece and she slotted it in, her small fingers clumsy with the knob. The parrot whistled loudly at us as a red and white plastic egg clattered down and Suzanne retrieved her prize.

'Thank you, Mummy.' Her teeth glinted white as a wide smile spread across her face. She shook the plastic toy, holding it out for me to see. I handed her back her special penny and she pushed it into her dungaree pocket. The tears and disappointment gone, faith restored, she bounced beside me as we made our way home.

A quiet knock and our front door opened to reveal a bright-eyed clean-shaven Pete. Our neighbour had offered the use of his van and his own time to drive us up to John o'Groats. He looked more suited to early mornings than the rest of us. He started to cheerily carry the boxes and bags stacked in the hall, carefully squeezing past our silver-framed tandem.

Another knock on the door and two bleary-eyed men entered. There was a cheery 'Hello' from Martyn. 'Are you set then?' he asked as the bright lights of his camera burnt into my eyes waking me more fully. Suzanne sat curled up in the corner of the settee, a cushion lifted to her face whenever the camera turned towards her as it followed Mike, Luke and me carrying belongings to the car. Rebecca and Steven, their hair straggling wildly from sleep, sat at the other corner of the settee. Steven rubbed his lip with his comfort-nappy, his eyes blinking slowly as he tried to keep himself awake.

'You'll be able to go back to bed soon,' I said.

'I'm too excited to sleep,' said Rebecca. 'I might just stay up and watch telly before I go to school.'

'Don't be silly,' I said. 'It's miles too early. You'd be better off getting back to bed.'

Luke roamed into the living room. 'Is there any marmalade?' he asked. 'I need a marmalade butty before we go.'

'I'll make you one,' called Mike from the kitchen. I could hear him cluttering about in a vague attempt at locating the preserve. I shivered and pulled my fleece about me, the front door was wide open and the chilly morning air was cooling the house. I walked through to the kitchen and perched on the stool wrapping my hands round the warm mug of coffee and watching Luke munch his way through a round of sandwiches. Half-listening to the banter between him and Mike, I watched the activity in the small hall. Too small for Martyn and Ian as they crowded in trying to catch the atmosphere of the early start. I heard the door of the van shut with a bang and Pete appeared with a great grin on his face. 'We're all packed then?'

I wandered back into the living room to say goodbye to the kids. The lamp of the camera lighting my way, following me as I bent to kiss their cheeks. 'You be good for Dad then,' I said. 'I'll see you very soon.'

I stepped up into the van and sat myself on the bench seat between Pete and Luke. My legs cramped slightly, as I twisted myself into the space left amongst the belongings filling every inch of the van. We turned to wave goodbye to the shivering foursome stood on the drive and made our way out of the estate.

We headed northwards up the A1 and had travelled past Scotch Corner before the sky started to lighten. Driving along the quiet road, the fog hanging low shrouded the way ahead. Off into the unknown, unsure whether we'd be returning this way still cycling or whether the hills in the Grampians would find me out and halt our three weeks' cycling early.

At our lunch stop we had a rendezvous with Uncle Dick and my cousin Chris. They had made their own way up driving the motorhome that was to be their base for the next few weeks. They were in high spirits – their vehicle bearing the signs for Jane's Appeal had drawn plenty of attention on their journey from Leeds. They'd even been given breakfast on the house at one of their stops.

At last, after about eleven hours sat in a cramped position in the van, we reached our journey's end, a bleak brown-green landscape with few buildings. Either side of the road were two white inns. Parked outside one was a grey van with satellite dishes aloft. A cameraman swaddled in a padded jacket trained his camera on us as we pulled into the car park. My heart jumped nervously.

'Where are Dick and Chris?' Luke voiced my own anxious thought. 'We haven't passed them.' We looked at each other, the road had been narrow with steep drops on the right-hand side. My mouth was dry, my fingers tingled with dread. Pete drove round to the rear of the car park and there in all its glory was the Jane's Appeal vehicle. The coldness left me as blood rushed back to my face and limbs. I was relieved they were safe.

We started unloading suitcases and boxes from the van while Luke busied himself with some adjustments on the bike. Checking into the hotel, the landlord looked up from his reservations list and asked, 'So who's paying for all these other rooms?'

I was momentarily stumped and looked at him confused. 'What rooms?'

'Well you're Jane Tomlinson. What about all these other bookings for Jane Tomlinson?'

A frustrating conversation ensued, at the end of which the landlord seemed no clearer in his understanding that the other people – mostly journalists and their cameramen – had booked into his hotel because of me, not with me. But the main thing was I had a key in hand for my room.

The afternoon was drawing on and the sun was dropping. After depositing the luggage in our room, Luke and I pulled on our black fleecy hats to protect ourselves from the fierce wind and walked the short distance along the road to the sea. Walking along the jetty we looked out across the grey sea, the mass of water lifted into white peaks as the wind caught it, blowing spray up on to the stone jetty. We sat with our legs hanging over the edge, glad to be away from the others, startled at the number of media folk who had appeared as if out of the woodwork. Awed by what we were to undertake the next day, we sat in contemplative silence until the cold made us stand and move away from the water's edge.

CHAPTER 2

March 2003

JANE

Waking early the next morning I left Luke sleeping and stood outside our room watching the sky turn pink as the golden edge of the sun erupted in the distance. Washing the bleak landscape with colour, it turned the grass golden and then green.

It was too early to warm myself by the first light and so I limped back into the room. My tendons and muscles were tight and it was painful to put my heels to the floor. The hot water spluttered from the taps as the bath slowly filled and I lowered myself in watching the white of my legs turn red but feeling my calves relax slightly.

Breakfast was a subdued affair. As people

around us tucked into cholesterol-laden fried eggs and bacon, I could only face scrambled eggs. My legs felt leaden and even sitting down my ankles were sore.

Luke finished his meal and was soon outside making last-minute adjustments to the bike. The satellite navigation system was attached, along with the maps for the day. My role was the navigator and, as any tandem rider knows, the stoker. Luke at the front was the pilot. After hooking the heavy panniers on to the rear, Luke stood astride the bike waiting for me to climb on. I readied my left foot on to the cage of the pedal and we set off slowly to the start line.

We had barely turned the pedals before we reached the white building with its grey spiked roof. It was the John o'Groats Hotel. We had registered the start of our journey in the record book at the public bar the day before and had been given a card to be filled in along the way so that Luke and I could be official 'end to enders'. Our journey from the most north-easterly inhabited corner of Britain to the south-westerly tip is made by around 4000 people every year and covers the greatest distance between two points on the British Isles.

As we wheeled the bike behind the official white start/finish line my nerves calmed and now it was heady exhilaration that left my body feeling light. My legs were sore but now that didn't matter. We were just about to start our journey and the next three weeks would be such an adventure – roads through parts of Britain I had never travelled, towns which were only names on motorway signs to be visited. I put my arm up on to Luke's shoulder.

'Are you ready for this?' he said.

I set the GPS system and nodded at his back. 'Yes.'

'Foot up then.' I raised my left foot in the pedal. We pushed down together and placed our right feet into the pedals as they reached the top of their arc. This was it. I could hear the laughter and lightness in Luke's voice, replacing the tension we'd both felt earlier. The silver bike moved quietly forward, pushed on by the steady movement of our black clad legs. We had twenty days' cycling ahead of us. I lifted my head from looking at the map and gazed around me at the quiet greenness, unable to keep the smile across my face from widening.

The road was quiet and we saw little traffic as we travelled parallel to the ragged northern coast past Gills Bay, where we could just make out an island in the near distance. The farmlands surrounding us held low scrubby grass and we gazed around quietly lost in our own worlds. Our legs turned with the quick synchronicity of the pedals as Dick and Chris swept past us in the support vehicle, beeping the horns and winding down the window to yell encouragement.

About one and a half hours after starting, we pulled up into a car park in Castletown and Chris opened the door of the motorhome. 'I've made you a cuppa,' he said and held a steaming mug out to each of us. I held the mug, blowing the steam and looking across the bay to Dunnet Head – the most northerly part of the British mainland.

The gentle stretching of my legs during our short tea break eased the cramp and, as we set off once more, I felt more confident of finishing the day without too much stress on my body.

But as we reached Thurso and headed west, the rolling hills turned into steep climbs. None of them were very great but as they rose up and out of the small towns, the gradient dramatically increased and we breathlessly cranked up the road that hugged the sea. Looking back on a spectacular view of the blue ocean, I lost my concentration for a second and had to turn my thoughts once more to the hard physical effort. Push two three, push two three – my legs stung as we reached the top and Luke and I panted our way over another crest, swooping down the hill. Luke steered the bike down and round the steep bends and I watched him carefully, making sure I leant the right way with him.

At the bottom of the hill we passed a sign for Bettyhill. Straining once more up another hill, I could see the white walls of our stopping place, the Bettyhill Hotel, ahead. My hair was matted against my head and salt trails snaked their way down my face. Our first day's cycling was over.

Across the road from the hotel overlooking Farr Bay and the vast sandy Torrisdale Bay, I could make out bright sails moving through the white-capped waves. 'Can you see those people out there?' I asked Luke.

'They must be mad,' said Luke, shivering. 'How are your legs feeling?'

'I'm fine. I don't feel like I have just cycled over fifty miles.'

51

Bettyhill Hotel had seen much grander days but what it lacked in luxurious finish it made up for in homely feeling. The sitting room felt like it could belong in your grandparents' house. In fact, the fireplace looked very much like one I remembered from my childhood. The room we were shown into was a mishmash of accumulated furniture. The bathroom, although it adjoined the bedroom, could not be called en suite, and had a door opening into the corridor.

While Luke disappeared off to chat with Dick and Chris and make himself busy with some fixing-up type-jobs, I decided I'd have a bath. As I ran the hot water, looking forward to stretching my tired body out, I sneaked back into the bedroom and pulled the curtains shut. Pulling and tugging my clothes off I left them scattered on the floor and grabbed my wash bag and went into the bathroom and shut the door. As I took out my shampoo and soap I noticed a keyhole in the door leading to our bedroom and experienced a sharp, sinking feeling. My clothes and towel were in the bedroom and I'd just locked myself out.

I pulled back the bolt on the door leading to the corridor and peered out along its length. There was no one around. Scanning the bathroom, I looked for something to cover my naked body with but there was only a small hand towel. I held it up to myself. If I was very careful, it just about covered my bust to the tops of my thighs. Trying not to think about my rear view, I double-checked the door. No, I definitely couldn't get into my room.

'Damn,' I spat. I tiptoed along the corridor, as

if that would in some way make me invisible, and found another door to another bathroom which provided me with yet another hand towel which I slung over my shoulder to cover a little more of my body.

I stood, panic-stricken, wondering how on earth I was going to rectify this embarrassing situation. I was so tired that I couldn't envisage sitting in the bath waiting for Luke to reappear – and, anyway, he might be several hours. The thought of going downstairs and appearing at reception clad in just my two hand towels made my stomach somersault, but I was so desperate that I didn't entirely dismiss the thought.

Stood there nearly naked, I heard someone coming. A workman-like whistling drew closer. I shouted, 'Hello, is there somebody there?' running as delicately as I could down the corridor.

Around a corner appeared a huge dungaree-clad man, with a shock of carrot-coloured hair. His burly eyebrows were raised as he looked down at me.

'I've locked myself out of my room,' I said by way of explanation.

'You have, haven't you?' he replied, as his eyebrows raised once more.

'Do you think you can help?'

'I'm sure I can,' he said and tried the door. It wouldn't budge. But rather than head downstairs to the reception, he took out a screwdriver from his pocket and jemmied the lock.

'Thanks, you're a lifesaver.'

'Ermm,' was his reply and he turned and made his way back down the corridor.

I sat on my bed, recovering from the shock, and picked up my key and towels and returned to the bathroom. To make especially certain of not embarrassing myself further, I propped open the door to the bedroom with a chair.

The following morning our legs felt fresh – our training had obviously paid off – and we were ready for the slightly shorter journey that would take us from Bettyhill to Lairg. On the map, the profile of the ride showed just one main climb up to Crask Inn, not like the first day which had been very up and down.

At reception, as I checked out, my ginger-haired rescuer greeted me with a good morning, leaving me red-faced and speechless.

The road was quiet as we headed away from the coast. It narrowed down to single track with only passing places and the small towns of yesterday were replaced by a beautiful landscape. The road running alongside the bank of Loch Naver was a dream to cycle. We stopped at the western edge in the small village of Altnaharra. The twenty-five miles covered felt easy, and the inn looked inviting. We ordered coffee and sat outside, our breathing deep and relaxed as we looked back on the road.

We were glad of that break when we set off. The road narrowed again and climbed up and up. We settled into a slow steady rhythm, the black tarmac disappearing as the wheels hissed over it.

'How high are we?' Luke asked and I flicked the switch on the GPS system.

'Seven hundred feet, and we're still climbing.'

'I thought the profile showed about six hundred feet.'

We both looked up and saw the road rising again to what must surely be the summit. I focused on the stone building ahead and it grew sharper and more in focus. At last we were at the top. Our feet down on tarmac, our legs shaking with the effort, we dismounted and wheeled the bike to the roadside. Luke lifted the heavy rear wheel weighed down with the panniers over to rest against the ornate milepost sign. Its two arms spread, it looked like a Celtic cross, black iron with symbols. With a curved smooth appearance, it fitted the landscape.

We sat on the roadside, sharp grasses penetrating our thin lycra as we rested. A tall gangling man walked over from the Crask Inn opposite. He was wearing a shapeless sweater. 'You'll be cycling the John o'Groats to Land's End route?' he asked.

We were surprised to hear a Yorkshire accent. 'Yes,' Luke answered.

'Aye. We get a lot of folks past here on their way,' he replied. 'It's a long old hill that one.'

'Tell us about it,' I said, still sprawled on the kerbside.

Luke wandered off with him and returned with a glass of dark swirling ale.

'It's good stuff this. You want to try it.' He passed the glass over and I took a long mouthful. The full malty taste of a cask-brewed ale hit my taste buds. It was good beer, a shame we still had another fifteen miles to cycle or else I would have joined Luke in a drink. I stuck to my water and watched as he chatted with this stranger telling him about our ride. He took Luke's glass and we readied ourselves to cycle into Lairg.

'Here take this.' Our host had appeared again and thrust a five pound note into my hand. 'You're doing a grand job.'

'Thanks. You didn't need to.' I gestured at the money.

'Every little helps,' he replied.

I thrust the note into the back pocket of my waterproof and Luke and I smiled and waved as we slowly started our descent. Loch Shin was a welcome sight an hour later and we cycled the last few miles towards our lodgings for the night. A small house, it was deceptively large inside with windows that overlooked the water. I showered and washed my cycling gear, wringing it out and hanging it in the shower cubicle to dry.

While Luke washed, I walked into the town and crossed a small bridge that took me to a sprawling wooded area. I shuffled through the fallen needles, the sharp smell of pine hitting the back of my nostrils. The sign said it was the Falls Shin, and although I didn't find them, I did enjoy the quiet solitude of the woods. There were carved trees in clearings. It was strange to think how the landscape we had travelled through must have changed. Thriving small communities disappearing when the land was turned over to grazing for sheep in the brutal Highland Clearances in the early 1800s. A simple phrase that belied the massacres and what would nowadays would be called ethnic cleansing.

I sat with my legs stretched out, enjoying the tranquillity. All the cycling was defining the muscles in my legs but made walking seem harder; the strain on my thighs made me turn back.

Back at the bed and breakfast, I rested. My bed was warm and comfortable and nestled under the quilt it was a wrench to rise to find somewhere to eat for the night. But our hunger lead us to the Nip Inn and the good food fuelled us for the next day.

Luke and I had been looking forward to a day of no hills, but the road to Inverness was a weary one. No hills meant no tortuous climbs, but it also meant no thrilling free rides downhill. It was just a slow slog on and on – small town after small town. The spectacular lonely moors through to Alness were replaced by the more drab towns of Dingwall and Beauly. As the day wore on, my navigating skills became questionable and I could hear Luke curse as he selected the wrong gear, my legs jerking as the mechanics threw our tired legs forward. The quickest route would have been down the A9, but the road looked too busy. The smaller roads were quieter with less traffic but the monotony of the day was staring to grind us down. Still it was a relief to reach Inverness. The McDougall Clansman Inn certainly deserved its name. The tartan floor carpeting was a novel patriotic gesture.

After such a long day I was despondent at finding only a shower in the room and no bath. I returned to reception to ask whether there was a bath in the entire hotel. After ignoring me for a long time, the receptionist took me upstairs and showed me a deserted bathroom, turned over to storage. The room was crammed full of broken items, the stained bath full of debris. Still, I was undeterred.

After clearing the bath of rubbish I enjoyed a long, hot soak. I had just dressed myself when Luke knocked on the door. 'Are you decent?' he said. He was grinning. 'Come and look at this.'

I followed him down the grand sweeping staircase. He opened the door to the room were we had stowed the bike and showed me the bathwater cascading through.

'That will be why they don't use the bathroom any more,' I said. The man who had been so slow to respond to me at reception was moving at some speed now as he shifted a bucket to catch the water.

'I'm glad I didn't know about that earlier,' I said. 'It might have spoiled my relaxation.'

That night was one punctuated by the battle cries of two opposing sets of football fans. Inverness had been home to Celtic that day and screams and blood-curdling threats rose from the pitched battles in the streets below.

I scratched at myself the next day. The bed had been lumpy and the sheets harsh. There had been a hearty bowl of porridge as well as the usual fry-up, which helped set me up for the day. We had covered 170 miles so far, and the hills had been useful practice for the fiercest climbs of the journey.

MIKE

Steven's school badge was not the only thing

58

adorning his grey school jumper. Although it was only Monday afternoon, there were remnants of his dinner staring out from his chest and I guessed that by Friday it would resemble a patchwork quilt of stains. He looked tired, his eyes slightly bloodshot, shoulders hunched.

'Do you want to see Mum on the telly tonight?' I leant over the car seat to study his response but he looked at me and said nothing. Although there was no coverage on Sky because they'd gone on to twenty-four-hour war coverage, Yorkshire TV were running updates at morning and night, usually with a live interview with Jane.

'Well?' I asked.

'Do I have to?'

'Well, I'd like to see her. Don't you want to?'

'Too boring,' he said, no trace of emotion in his voice.

'Oh.'

Within a couple of minutes we were home. As I opened the door my ears were assaulted by cacophonous sounds, which seemed to be coming from every room. I shouted 'Hello' but was not surprised when no response came. Steven brushed past me, closely followed by Morris, one of our two cats. Steven discarded his shoes and fleece in the middle of the floor.

'Hang them up, Steven.' He made a half-hearted attempt and I finished it off for him. My entrance to the kitchen was barred by Suzanne, who was kneeling on the floor putting some laundry in the washing machine. 'I'll do that, Suzanne,' I said.

'You what?'

I reached across, unplugging her ghetto blaster that was blaring out the latest Gomez track, but the void was filled by the shrieking laughter from *Friends* on the TV in the living room.

'Turn that down, Becca!' I looked through the porthole window in the washing machine. 'Suzanne, you can't just put three items in there. It's not economical.'

'You can't mix colours.'

'Well, just leave them until next weekend, when we'll have a full load.'

'I want my red top for tomorrow though.'

I sighed. 'It would be cheaper to buy a new one. Anyway your mum said I was to do the washing.' Her face frowned in a manner only a sulky teenager can perfect. 'Look, the lids should be on the pans otherwise the kitchen will get steamed up,' I said, pushing past her to get to the cooker. 'And take your shoes off in the house.'

'Oh that's it, come in and take it out on me because you've had a bad day at work,' she snapped before storming off.

'Becca, turn that bloody telly down,' I yelled.

'Dad I'm hungry.' I looked down at Steven whose hand was tentatively reaching towards the biscuit jar.

'What did you have for dinner?' I asked.

'Not telling you,' he said and grabbed a biscuit. I looked outside towards the vivid colours of Jane's tulips in the garden – orange, violet, white – they brightened my disposition. Turning back I noticed a mug of steaming tea. Suzanne's good intentions couldn't be faulted. Looking around, the kitchen work surfaces required clearing, the

60

table setting, the dryer emptying, Steven needed to be fed and our tea to be finished. I caught myself and thought, apologise.

'Dad the phone's ringing,' Steven shouted.

Passing the living-room door I called out, 'For god's sake, Becca, turn that bloody telly down.'

'Okay.'

'No it's not bloody okay, you haven't lifted a finger. Suzanne, can you help while sulking please? Hello,' I barked.

'Hi, love, are you all right?' Jane's voice seemed unnaturally calm.

'No, Becca's being a pain, Suzanne's sulking and Steven's tired.' I knew immediately I sounded churlish and spoilt.

'Oh well, you'll just have to deal with it as you would see fit. You are the adult after all.' Maybe it was just me, but Jane seemed a little disappointed not to be a part of our minor domestic.

'How was today?' I asked.

'Okay,' she said. 'We were all tired after the noise of last night. I'll have to go, I've got a live interview to do in twenty minutes for ITV. What time should I ring later?'

'Half eight after Steven's in bed.'

As I was replacing the receiver, Steven ran from the living room 'Dad, your mobile.' I ran to collect it, an interview request for Jane. Real Radio. As we finished talking I noticed a faint burning smell from the kitchen. Dashing over to the hob, I slipped on the lino causing my right leg to jar at the knee. Reaching for the pan lid, I flinched as my fingers burnt on the metal. The lid went crashing on to the hob, noisily echoing around the kitchen.

'Dad, the phone!' Becca shouted from the living room, not moving a muscle. I dashed to the hall. The phone's display read 'international'.

'Suzanne, sort the tea; it's burning. Come on, now,' I urged. Lifting the receiver there was a familiar nano-second delay of the dreaded cold-call from a double glazing centre or patio vendor.

'Is that Mr Tomlinson, the homeowner?' said a voice in broken English.

'No.' I slammed the phone down, hitting the receiver, and it bounced and landed perfectly on the second attempt. I stared at it menacingly. 'Suzanne, now!'

The phone rang again displaying 'Number withheld' on the caller ID.

'What?' I barked.

'Is that Mike Tomlinson?' I had an overwhelming urge to issue a string of obscenities but bit my tongue.

'Yes,' I said, barely disguising my irritation.

'Are you the husband of Jane Tomlinson who is cycling in Scotland?'

'Yes. Excuse me a second,' I placed the receiver on the settle. Steven was in tears on the floor.

'What's up?' I asked.

He sniffled, 'Becca.'

'Well, it was the adverts,' Rebecca said. I looked across at the telly where a puerile pop band were formation-dancing to supermarket music.

'Even so, Becca, no one should be subjected to that. Turn it back.' The beginnings of a migraine were starting to form; I applied pressure to my temple and lifted the phone, 'Sorry, how can I help?'

'I am phoning on behalf of the Lord Lieutenant of West Yorkshire who wondered whether Jane would be interested in being nominated for an honour in the Queen's Birthday Honours List. It would either be an MBE or an OBE.'

I paused, momentarily caught off-guard, and it took me a few seconds to process the information. 'Err, well, it's never crossed her mind. Err, I don't know.' I gave it a moment's thought and then added, 'Well, yes, I'm sure she'd be delighted.'

'Good. Well with what she's doing and has achieved she would be a deserving recipient. Time is against us though; we need to have the forms submitted by Thursday. Jane would need to be nominated by someone, but it's just a formality. Would you be so kind as to document her achievements, a timeline and write a formal nomination letter?' I pondered the request. 'Can I come and collect them all tonight?'

'Ermm, I don't know.'

'Well, if it's not convenient I could call round tomorrow but it'll be probably too late to post.'

'It's not that I'm unhappy to do the timeline. However, I'm not prepared to nominate her. That should come from someone who is not connected with us. If she really does deserve an honour, the nomination should come from other people.'

'Oh, for all she's done she definitely deserves the award.'

'Sorry, I don't want to be difficult, but I'm just not prepared to nominate her myself.'

'It is just a formality.'

'I hear what you're saying but I still don't want to nominate her for an award.'

'Is there anyone you feel who could write such a letter? A charity, someone you've worked with? Someone in the media?'

'I'm sure there is, though it's not something I think that I should be involved in. I'm sorry but if it's reliant on me getting the nomination for her she'll have to go without.'

He paused before conceding that he understood my position. 'I'll resolve the nomination issue if you can get the timeline done,' he said. 'I'll pop round in an hour to collect it.'

I replaced the receiver. 'Shit, shit, shit,' I muttered opening the kitchen door. 'Suzanne, pop my tea in the oven, I need to do a job first.' She threw a disgusted look and turned her back on me. For thirty minutes I drafted and redrafted the timeline. Although I wasn't prepared to nominate Jane, I was immensely proud that the Lord Lieutenant's office could consider her worthy of such an award and I wanted the document to be perfect. Time was disappearing and it began to feel like the pressure of writing an exam essay. A shadow from the hall light indicated Suzanne had come in the front room-cum-office.

'Are you all right?' she said.

'Yes.'

'Your tea's ruined.'

'Yes, Mum.'

'Don't take the piss. What are you doing?'

'Can't say. Will you leave me alone so I can get it finished though?'

'Whooahh, sorry.'

I barely saw the children before they went to bed. Suzanne fitted the role of a substitute mum perfectly, bathing and getting Steven ready for bed. By the time the timeline was done, correspondence answered and e-mails sent to local newspapers and radio stations in the areas that Jane was to visit over the next three days, it was half past one in the morning. I caught sight of myself in the mirror – my eyes were bloodshot and sore.

Within five minutes I was in bed but was unable to relax from the stress and adrenalin of the last few hours. I tossed and turned. Eventually, the living-room clock, chiming hourly until six o'clock, prompted me to get up to continue the work of last night.

As soon as I rose I felt more relaxed knowing that I could get a couple of hours work done before I needed to go to the office. As a consequence, the overwhelming desire to sleep overtook me.

JANE

Inverness was busy the next morning as we set off and my navigating skills were severely questioned. In the end we had some help from a friendly traffic warden – now there's three words not used together very often. I followed the direction in which his hand was gesturing.

'Down to the first set of traffic lights, and bear left. Ignore the signs for Inverness but bear straight on until you come to the second roundabout.' He carried on with his complicated explanation of how to leave Inverness and we turned the bike and waited for a gap in which to set off. His goodwill even extended to holding up the traffic and we set off optimistically in the direction he'd waved. Looking back as we waited at the first set of traffic lights he pointed his hand right and gave us the thumbs up. Half-turned in my saddle I waved my thanks.

'Now which set of lights do we go left at?' I asked Luke.

'I don't know. I wasn't listening,' he replied.

'Oh. Well if we ignore this next junction.' I faltered, my head was struggling with lefts and rights but I knew we had a climb out of the city so I figured we were headed right. 'That's the A9,' I shouted unable to disguise my glee. 'Yep, and this is the road that goes past Culloden.' Confident of my directions now and finding myself on the map, I relaxed.

The road surface was ill-maintained and we ground out the miles. I felt tired, and my legs didn't seem to be moving with ease. I was finding it hard to shake off a despondency that had crept over me yesterday. The long dreary ride had been made even more depressing after seeing a well-wisher in one of the many small towns.

'It's good to see you,' she had said. I shook her hand and smiled. 'You know, I was like you. I had surgery and radiotherapy. I didn't need chemo though, thank goodness.'

'Oh, that's good, and how are you now?' I asked.

'Oh I'm one of the lucky ones, I've been fine since. It's five years now and it's all behind me.'

I looked at her, dressed up for Sunday dinner;

her silver hair brushed, the pearls at her neck contrasting with the dark sweater.

'Oh, I'm so glad,' I said and she shook my hand once more and we set off again. As we followed the road out of town I couldn't stop the tears rolling down my cheeks.

'Come on, girl,' Luke said. 'I don't think she quite realised how that came out.'

I sniffled along for another couple of miles before I started to feel less gloomy. But her words had stayed with me. Why wasn't I 'one of the lucky ones'? Why had my cancer spread? Those thoughts had stayed with me for the rest of the day and weighed down on me as we cycled along the empty moorlands.

We had left the cars and noise of Inverness behind us. It was quiet and still as we cycled through the area of the battlefields, so many deaths here. The sense of the spirits of the many people who had visited this isolated place remained with us as we climbed the hills up to the high moorlands. It clung to us for many more miles and only seemed to leave us as we whooped and screeched on a frantic downhill into Bridge of Dulsie.

The tight corners and steep descent concentrated our minds and left us stopping just short of a small humpback bridge that crossed the River Findhorn. I brushed my hand through my short hair raking the damp ends away from my face, pushing away the tiredness. The last few moments of the drop down to the narrow strip of water had lifted our mood. As we sat perched on stones surrounded by sheep and ate sandwiches, our faces were pink with the exertions of the morning. Laughing, I pushed myself to my feet, holding my lunch high up away from the animals' long black noses before stuffing it into my mouth.

The short day seemed hard on our legs and we needed to stop and eat regularly to keep the pace over the ever increasing slopes. Maybe it was the thought of the monstrous climbs to come through the Grampians and the Lecht Pass, highest point on the trip, which made the gloom of the previous day descend on us once more. It made the bike's load seem heavier and left us feeling lethargic.

We knew we were due to stop in a bed and breakfast over the Bank of Scotland in Grantown-on-Spey. We were surprised to see that the bank was open for business. Customers came and went all afternoon.

More pleasing was my sumptuous bed and the spacious room. Our host apologised to us that we didn't have our own bathroom, but the white fluffy robes more than made up for the tiny inconvenience. I sat immersed in sweet smelling water listening to the hiss of the hot-water system and felt myself relaxing.

After the bustle of Inverness, the quiet grandness of Grantown-on-Spey was refreshing, and I walked down the main street stopping to look through the windows. I stepped into the bookshop and browsed through the eclectic collection, finding so many travel and gardening books I couldn't possibly decide which one to buy. So I left them all.

Luke was busy with minor adjustments to the intricate gears of the tandem when I returned.

When he had finished fine tuning the machine he washed, removing the oil from the bike and the grime from the road. We couldn't face another evening of pub food so went for the healthy option of fish and chips instead, wrapped up and smelling of vinegar, from the little chippy round the corner.

It was hard to rouse myself the next morning, the bed felt too inviting, the covers nestled round me too warm to leave. A small tinge of light from the sun fell through the heavily draped windows and I threw back the covers and pulled myself out of bed, groaning at the thought of putting on my cycling shorts yet again. They were still damp from the day before and I shuddered as they made contact with my legs. At least my top was dry. I pulled the brush through my unruly shock of hair and I eased the blue and red knee supports up my legs. I'd need them for the climbs today.

The coffee was too good to turn down a second cup, but we couldn't put off the day's hard climbing any longer. Luke dragged my suitcase downstairs while I threw some supplies into the pannier. Our support vehicle with Dick and Chris had been meeting our needs on the road with drinks and Chris made sandwiches each day. Every day it was a surprise to see what ingredients had been placed between the bread. Would it be tuna and cheese or peanut butter and cheese today I wondered?

The skies were overcast, the day was much cooler and Luke and I were pleased to be putting on extra layers – today was a day of climbs.

Starting at 9 a.m. we left Grantown-on-Spey.

We coasted down towards the River Spey and then started the climbs. With the Hills of Cromdale to our left we pushed upwards before an exhilarating downhill to the Bridge of Brown.

I could imagine the grin on Luke's face as he whooped on the downhills. As we neared the bottom of a particularly steep and fast downhill, he turned to me and asked, 'How scary was that?'

It was barely 10 a.m. when we climbed off the bike at Tomintoul and sat on benches that were placed around the green. Our fingers were cold from the air rushing by us and we warmed them with mugs of coffee from Chris. We didn't stop too long, the climbs had warmed our bodies and they were quickly chilling as we sat. I shivered as I pulled on my helmet and fastened it below my chin. The next climb would be very demanding – one and a half thousand feet up to Lecht Pass.

The road started to climb only gradually and the sensation of pushing ourselves, of pushing the bike on, was satisfying. When we saw the road soar up ahead of us, I lowered my eyes, ignoring the climb. Beside the road were dirty patches of snow, pockets filling where the sun hadn't shone. I let go of the handlebars and pulled down the zip of my coat. Sweat slid down the side of my face and I groaned as my legs started to burn.

Determined not to set our feet down till we reached the top, we forced our legs round. I could hear Luke exhaling sharply, see his body push from side to side ahead of me as we set ourselves against the hill. The rhythm was good and the road passed under our wheels. I felt like the pass was pulling us forward, till at last we reached the summit. The snow huts and lodges looked abandoned, in season neither for snow pursuits nor for walking.

We sat huddled in the motorhome for lunch. An unexpected treat, the taste was difficult to analyse. I opened the sandwich to examine the filling, to see what the explanation for the assault on my taste-buds was. Cheese, peanut butter and marmite. A hideously revolting combination to put between slices of bread, but I was too hungry and tired to bother making anything different so I ate it anyway.

After lunch, the downhill when we got on the bike was rapid, but soon forgotten in the next climb out of Cock Bridge and the following one after that. The road seemed to last for ever through the grounds of Balmoral Castle, the twists and turns not coming close to disguising the gradient leading up to Braemar. We pushed and pushed until at last Luke and I could take no more cycling, our legs refusing to turn. Even the knowledge that we were just two miles from our destination couldn't drive us on any further and we sat disconsolately at the roadside, shovelling some more food in our mouths, hoping it would give us a boost. While we sat there against the stone wall, our feet pushing around the leaf mould from the winter, we looked about us. The darkening gloom of the wooded road suited our mood.

The relief of just five minutes without pedalling allowed us to climb back on the bike looking forward to the last couple of miles, enjoying the loneliness of the road and eventually the view of Braemar Castle's splendid grandeur as we rounded the turn to arrive in the town.

The stylish furnishings of Bank House from the previous day were followed by another warm and welcoming bed and breakfast at Callater Lodge. Greeted with coffee and biscuits and a bath and wrapped with warm towels I started to feel the exertions of the day leave my legs and back.

The next day was calm as we set off. It was our last day in the Grampian Mountains and we had one long climb to begin. There were more small climbs but much of the day was spent in easy downhill sections as we descended towards Perth. We found our hotel by the railway station. Dick and Chris were sitting in the car park waiting to drive off in hope of finding a caravan showroom or at least somewhere that would fix the niggling small leak in the shower and toilet area of the motorhome.

I dragged my suitcase down the steps off the van and Luke and I headed by car towards Perth Airport. I had been dreading the drive back to Leeds for my chemotherapy treatment, so when Darren Stubbs of Consort Homes – with the help of Leeds Flying School – offered me return flights in a small plane I jumped at the chance. Sitting outside watching the planes land and seeing the minute size of the aircraft, I began to feel a quivering in my stomach. My fists tightened round the strap of my bag.

Darren helped me step up on to the wing and into the aircraft. 'Here, you need to fasten these,' Darren said, as he located the straps that went over my shoulders and across my lap. 'There's a headset there.' I put it on and Darren's voice came through the padded earphones. 'Can you hear me okay?'

We set off down the runway. It was like being in a very fast, very small, very noisy car. The tarmac bumped under us. It seemed a long moment until the plane lifted and the bumping was substituted by the strange sensation of a misplaced metal body forcing its way through the air. It was a ludicrous thing to be in such a small place travelling through the air, the propellers turning so they were no more than a blur, the air rushing under the wings at such a speed to allow us to continue suspended above the earth.

'Hi,' said Nikki, a representative from Cancer Research. She put her arm around me and squeezed my shoulder. 'What was the flight like?'

'It was great,' I replied, 'like being in a sports car, only the view was better.'

'How's the cycling going?' Nikki asked.

'Okay, but it will be good to have a day off the bike.'

'What, even if it's to have chemo?'

'Well, it's not ideal, but it is still a rest.'

After the aircraft the car journey home from Leeds Bradford Airport seemed pedestrian, but still it was a refreshing change from cycling along at 15 m.p.h.

I was tired and found the house busy and noisy after so much solitude. Suzanne and Becca bickered about tidying the kitchen. Steven was tired from his day at school.

I had to filter out some sounds to talk to Mike and the kids. Still they found me distant, but it wasn't that I didn't want to talk to them, rather that my senses were bombarded and overloaded. I took the opportunity of using the washing machine. I knew that on my return with a bag full of freshly laundered kit Luke would be truly envious.

The evening passed quickly and I fell into bed exhausted. Even at home I was still living out of a suitcase, as I was travelling back to Perth straight after my chemo the next day.

After chemo I sat at the airport sucking sweets as we waited for the air clearance for our route. Darren handed me a bag to be sick in. 'Don't forget to take your headphones off,' he said. 'We don't want to listen to you if you're ill.'

I nodded nervously, unsure if my stomach would be settled on the return flight. Chemo made me nauseous, but I usually managed not to vomit. The journey back was at 4500 feet, just below cloud level, so I could make out the landscape we would be passing through in the next few days. I was even able to pick out some of the climbs that lay ahead of us. We passed several cities which were easy to identify by the brown-grey smog hanging over the area.

Back at Perth I hugged Darren and thanked him. I was glad I'd taken the opportunity, it was an experience I would never have had otherwise.

Luke looked tired and in need of a coffee. So, when I had stowed my bag in the hotel room, we walked into Perth to the Willow Café and sat enjoying a milky coffee. I ordered some soup, hoping it would settle my still lurching stomach, and could barely look at Luke's haggis sandwich.

He, however, ate it with relish, having examined the filling with great interest before eating it.

Sitting there, in the warmth of the café, I felt complete despair at the thought of cycling the next day. Not that I wasn't looking forward to the rest of the journey, it was just that it would have been good to sit in one place for a day or two before continuing on our way. But the schedule had to be kept to.

Back at our spacious room Luke and I sat on our beds and looked at each other.

'It's not far tomorrow,' I said, tracing my finger over the following day's route on the map. 'I still don't fancy it though.'

'I know what you mean.' Then Luke's face lit up, his eyes twinkling. 'I tell you what, the bathroom is enormous.'

'Yes?' I said, questioningly.

'Well, do you fancy helping me wash the bike in it? It could do with some cleaning to get the muck off.'

'Oh, go on then.' We sneaked downstairs and retrieved our bike from the storeroom, giggling as we manoeuvred it round the narrow staircase, trying to hide from the hotel staff. We got to the top of the stairs, only to recognise the folly of our plan. The bathroom might be big enough, but the hall was way too narrow. The angle was too sharp. Luke looked rather stumped and sat looking at the door.

'No problem,' he said after a few seconds as he stood the bike up on its hind wheel and pushed it through the tall door. We used some of the complimentary shampoo to sponge the bike off and then showered the suds away. Lifting the bike free, Luke turned the pedals and showered me with greasy water.

'Oi!' I cried. Then, 'Oh, look at that!' As the water gurgled down the drain it left the white enamelled bath black with grime. Greasy grime that didn't shift with the shower.

'It'll be right,' said Luke. We looked at each other and laughed. It was the first time we had laughed together that day.

Luke bucked the bike up and back through to the bedroom and we upturned it on to its handlebars and saddles. It looked denuded without its panniers and handlebar bag – a strange steed with its pedals circling slowly, clicking quietly and fruitlessly. I took some body scrub through to the bathroom and started rubbing it into the black rings around the bath. It took some time and while Luke fine-tuned the gears, fixing the slip which had been irritating us the last cycling day, I cleaned the bath out. It was by no means sparkling, but it was at least acceptable, and no longer looked as if a whole shift of miners had bathed in it.

We had no time for any decent breakfast the following morning. Not wanting to dally too long, we shovelled a currant teacake down and got on the road. The chill had brought mist. It was a day of cycling in and out of damp clinging areas. Passing under and over the motorways it was amazing that within just several hundred yards of leaving them behind, the sound was deadened. The mist turned into rolling dense fog, settling over the Forth Road Bridge as we cycled alongside the traffic. Even there, the noise was eerily muffled by the fog. The sun, which we had seen now and then briefly, fought and lost the battle to penetrate the dense fog.

We turned right after the bridge looking for the centuries-old Hawes Inn, reputed to be haunted. Pulling up outside, we secured the tandem to some railings and entered a brightly lit pub.

'That was a shorter day than I thought,' I said to Luke. 'It's a shame we can't see the bridge. Maybe the fog will lift later.'

'What time did you say Mike was arriving?'

'Oh, about fiveish I think,' I replied.

MIKE

Mist shrouded the Forth Road Bridge so that the metal frame promised a tantalising trip to the sky. Only the hum of traffic spoilt the tranquillity and then to the right an increasing rhythmic tapping, like water dripping into an empty plastic sink, indicated a commuter train leaving the city.

Steven and I dangled our legs over a wooden jetty listening to the water lap against the shale. Edinburgh was only eight miles to the east, and although I'd anticipated driving there to show Steven the castle, it was futile as we'd see nothing.

We'd arrived with Rebecca and Luke's 12-year-old daughter, Sue, thirty minutes earlier after a tedious six-hour drive from Leeds. Jane initially seemed thrilled to see us all, hugging us and enthusiastically regaling us with stories and bombarding us with questions about home. Soon, however, it was clear she was frustrated by us being there as we were hindering her from continuing her daily routine.

Although Jane had been in Leeds on Tuesday and Wednesday to have chemotherapy we had parted on poor terms. Jane hadn't been keen on my plan for her to fly home in a two-seater plane, thinking a car would be quicker. I was irritated at her apparent thoughtlessness at the trouble we'd gone to on her behalf. Even in the telephone conversations we shared, there had been a staccato rhythm to our chat and long pregnant pauses until the next insult could be traded. It was understandable. We were both under enormous pressure and were lacking in our usual patience.

Jane had been remarkably chirpy on her home trip when not irritated by me, but the in-jokes and general bonhomie that she had shared with her accompanying TV crews had left me and the children feeling a little cold – not to mention left out.

To add to the tense atmosphere, while Jane was at home, we'd discovered that a tabloid reporter was trying to investigate whether Jane was actually cycling all the way. It was a ridiculous notion – which if true would have required collusion with two TV crews – but the thought that it could even be considered by the papers put us all on the defensive.

On Jane's first day away I had attended the funeral of a friend Wendy who'd died of cancer. Many friendships are forged through shared circumstances, school, university and work, and so I suppose it's natural that when health issues mean frequent and regular visits to hospitals similar friendships are made. That's how I met Wendy and John, in the outpatients' waiting area of St James's Hospital one Tuesday afternoon. Of course, the disadvantage of an oncology-department-formed friendship is that it's rarely permanent and to watch the deterioration of fellow patients, the increased pain, slowing of speech and reduced mobility, is to gaze into the crystal ball of your own life.

On this occasion, the deterioration in Wendy's breast cancer had been rapid, a fast-forward of what we ourselves would be going through at some point in time. Jane's medical background meant she was able to predict Wendy's rapid loss of health and although I was aware that Jane's knowledge was substantial, it had still taken me by surprise. For the first time – although I'd probably already subconsciously known – I'd realised that Jane could translate her own symptoms into her own prognosis. She'd know when the end would be near.

Receiving the terminal diagnosis was, from day one, a palliative care journey. On that same day, ladies of differing age were given similar diagnoses and so they began on the same journey to the same destination. The only difference was how long it was going to take each one to reach it.

For some, treatment would delay their disease and, certainly, in the oncology departments there was never any sense of jealousy from the other patients – just a vicarious sense of pleasure that someone's life expectancy has been extended. That joy was always multiplied when the patient was younger – it meant they would be able to see a little more of their youth.

The following morning, Jane and Luke had suggested I cycled the second half of the day with them rather than the whole day. This was probably as a result of my rather difficult mood. It suited Steven especially well as it meant he could travel in the motorhome; something he'd been nagging me about since he knew we had one.

Being in the support crew is excruciatingly tedious – constantly leapfrogging the tandem only to watch it go past in a matter of seconds. The novelty of seeing two cyclists clad in luminous yellow ride past you soon wears off. And it was becoming increasingly clear that it had the same effect on Jane and Luke.

'Will you get out of the fucking way in future?' Jane said to me when they took the first break. On narrow roads, the motorhome had been quite an obstacle. I, of course, dealt with her in a grown-up and responsible manner.

'Fuck off, you miserable cow,' I spat, before skulking off like a scolded schoolboy.

Luke assembled my bike after dinner. With only two weeks to go before the marathon, I should have been in peak condition but my heart pounded just getting my leg over the crossbar. I'd like to say I'd been diligent with the marathon training, but the bike ride had soaked up all available time. Apart from a couple of short runs, the longest distance I'd attempted in the previous six weeks was fourteen miles. Attempted was the key word. I'd managed to run eight, walk two and jib on the last four.

For the first three miles of the ride I stayed with the tandem, out of the saddle and dancing on the pedals during the climbs. Slowly, however, the gap between myself and the tandem grew – from 50 yards to 100 to 150 to 200 and then they were merely a dot on the distant hill. After thirty minutes they were only a faded memory. It was a depressing lonely afternoon. At one point I mistakenly dissected a golf course, attracting the attention of two old golfers who shouted: 'Get off and milk it' at me.

I'd expected abuse, but from two overweight geriatric golfers wearing matching pink jumpers, it was too much to take. By the time I'd reached the agreed resting place Jane and Luke were getting ready to set off again. The only consolation had been that my saddle had been changed quickly by Luke from a racing one to one that would accommodate the most obese of people. Even so my arse already felt like it had a tennis ball attached to each cheek.

By the time the day had finished in Jedburgh in the Scottish Borders it was past six o'clock. As I pulled up, Jane and Chris Kiddy from ITV were waiting for me.

'You look a touch flushed, Mike. Did you enjoy it?' Chris asked. I drew a deep breath.

'He's only done thirty-six out of the fifty-four miles,' Jane replied on my behalf. I drew another breath. With a monumental effort I put my leg over the handlebar. My tiredness forced the bike to shake and I momentarily lost balance.

'Come on, Mike, hurry up,' said Jane. 'It's late

and we're normally finished by mid-afternoon. I need a shower and something to eat – it's nearly dark.'

'Have some patience.'

'Patience! We've been waiting thirty minutes, get a grip.'

I could feel my clothes stick to my skin from sweat. I was cold, hungry and about to check into some low budget accommodation about as welcoming as a puncture.

Twenty-four hours later we were in Corbridge, a lovely town on a beautiful late Sunday afternoon. The sun was beating down and despite being late March it had a real May feel. Each pub had a throng of drinkers sitting outside. Jane and Luke were the first to finish for the day and by the way Jane was hobbling it hadn't been a pleasant time in the saddle. Even driving it hadn't been easy. I had driven down the corrugated A68 and it had been horrendous. The route's profile – which we had seen before the start of the ride – indicated that it would have climbs of 6600 feet which suggested that it would be the toughest climb of the trip, a notion quickly dismissed by everyone. Oh, how the maps hadn't lied.

Jane and Luke propped the tandem against the guesthouse wall, both had sunken cheeks and eyes glazed over.

'Are you all right?' I asked Jane. She stared past me at the revellers across the street. After waiting a respectable time I repeated the question.

'Not really. It was tough. You can't get enough momentum on the downhills to get any advantage on the uphills.'

'Where are Ian and Martyn?'

'Behind. Ian's been really struggling. He was thinking about giving up ten miles back.'

Jane looked momentarily vulnerable, on the precipice of dissolving into tears. The laughter from the pub crowd across the road seemed at odds with how we were feeling.

'Have you got any food or drink for us?' Jane asked. In truth I'd never given it a moment's thought.

'I've scoured the town but couldn't see anything you'd like.' Jane had removed her helmet, replacing it over the handlebars. She turned around and walked towards me, fists clenched, her body bulked by the cycling jacket. She moved forward purposefully with a look of irritation that would have put Ricky Hatton on his guard.

'You've not looked have you?' she demanded.

'Well, ermm,' I spluttered.

'Don't lie...' she said and I wondered what was coming next. 'Just give me a hug then.'

JANE

The next day as we headed out of Corbridge (minus Mike who had returned home again), the A68 continued on its roller coaster way and we tackled the relentless climbs up to blind summits followed by delightful downhills. We'd only been on the road for an hour and a half when the pedals turned freely and our momentum halted: the long gear cable had snapped.

I sat in the long grass by the side of the road

and marvelled at Luke's cool as he upended the bike. He hummed to himself as he checked the potential damage.

'No problem,' he said as he uncoiled a long, long cable. 'It's a good job I brought a spare.' From out of one of the panniers he brought a coiled loop and measured it up against the frayed edges of the snapped wire. The sun was out pensively as he threaded the wire and tightened it, running the bike through the gears, adjusting it till it was set for cycling.

We wheeled the bike to the top of the slope, the incline would have put too much pressure on the cable and we couldn't afford to have it snap again. Our legs raced round as we tried to catch up some time – we still had fifty miles more to cover that day and the hills didn't stop coming.

At last we reached the right exit on the A68 and we turned on to the old Roman route of Dere Street and pulled over. We had a small dance of satisfaction watching the lorries roar past towards Darlington and relief that we would no longer be part of that dreaded road, which – although it had saved us many miles – had nearly broken our spirits over the last day and a half.

The Romans had a reputation for building straight roads, ignoring the contours of the land, and Dere Street was no exception. You could imagine columns of Roman soldiers clattering along as they marched down the dead straightness that faced us. Each summit revealed another and yet more in the distance stretching on as far as we could see. I felt like weeping as I adjusted my bottom on the saddle, trying to find some comfort as my weight bore down through the pelvic bones. It was almost hypnotic watching Luke's legs, push-pulling the pedals up and round. I counted the strokes in my head and looked in front once more.

We crossed the A66 and, looking at my map, I could see we were just two miles from Scotch Corner. The journey to Richmond looked like it should take twenty minutes but the high-banked lanes hid the climbs ahead.

'Nearly there, Luke.'

'You've been saying that for ages.'

'No honestly,' I replied. 'When we get to Richmond I'm finding a bun shop.' I stopped talking as the hill steepened and my breathing became more ragged.

We pulled up at the large square surrounded by shops, and I left Luke chinwagging with Chris and went in search of some fancies. I leant wearily against the counter as I watched the woman box them up.

'Take your pick,' I said as I placed the box on the table in the motorhome and gratefully accepted the coffee placed in my hands by Chris.

'How much further?' Luke asked.

I looked at the map. 'I reckon about 10 miles.'

'I'm going to go on ahead,' said Chris. 'Oh, and Mark phoned. He says he'll see you tonight.'

My brother Mark had wanted to join us when we first started talking about the trip, and had settled on meeting up with us for one day. The thought of seeing him gave us renewed vigour to apply to the pedals and we set off once more.

My poor navigational skills and tired head made it hard to find the exit we needed but at last we came to the river and we were soon on the road out of Richmond heading towards Catterick Garrison. We came across signs for slow moving tanks and laughed – until we came alongside a slow moving tank.

At last, we arrived at Snape and the Castle Arms. We cycled round the back looking for Chris, but no white motorhome was evident. The doors to the pub were all locked, and there was a tall wall round the back of it with a locked gate. We sat on the waterlogged parking lot and I could have wept. I was so tired; all I wanted was to lie down.

'I've rung Chris. He's just down the road at the last town,' said Luke. 'He'll be here in a quarter of an hour.'

'Thank goodness for that. I just want to get changed.'

There was a celebratory atmosphere as we ate that night. Mark had arrived, the food was excellent and the beer was the Black Sheep Brewery's heavy dark brew. Full and feeling a little tipsy, Luke and I retired to our rooms.

Next morning, I could hear the wind and the rain before pulling back the drapes. At the window, fat drops spattered against the glass, and dry leaves rushed in circles madly round the enclosed garden. We shuddered as we pulled on extra layers. We had trained in sleet and snow so the damp didn't bother us, but we'd not had to cope with it yet on our ride.

The rain had lessened to a drizzle, the wind blowing it hard into our faces as we set off. The tiredness of the last few days was a distant memory, our legs lightened by the knowledge we would be home tonight. So as we flew down the road into Ripon, the wind seemed to change direction, pushing us down the road, rather than throwing stinging rain at us. We skirted Ripon and pulled up at the racecourse, shivering as our warm bodies cooled down quickly, waiting for Mark to appear.

When he appeared he shook his head free from the constraining helmet we had insisted he wear, and laughed. 'Where did you two disappear to?'

I knew there was no way Luke would have allowed Mark to pass us. But the bike had sung its sweet song over the tarmac that morning, and we hung low and turned our legs to the hum of the mechanism as we powered our way over small hills and whooshed through valleys.

As we cycled down the quiet lane with East Keswick to the right of us, Mark pushed his bike up the steepest of the hills that day. 'Right, that's me done with,' he said as he pulled off his helmet.

'Come on, you can keep going into Leeds,' Luke said.

'Nope, I've had a great day but I'm better off finishing now while I'm still enjoying it.' He laughed. 'I'm knackered. How have you two managed to get here? I can't believe it.'

'It gets easier,' I said. Luke raised his eyebrows.

The undulations of the road were familiar from all the training runs we'd done. The spears of yellow pushing upwards on the verges, still to burst into trumpets of daffodils, were a contrast to the deep blue-green of the swaying grasses over the hills. The white of the limestone faults was echoed by the dotted flocks of sheep.

The open fields and greens of golf courses became narrow stone-walled lanes as we cycled into the outskirts of north Leeds and headed towards Luke's house. The emblazoned support van was parked in all its glory outside. As we climbed off the bike, Mark opened the door.

'What took you so long?' he chortled loudly.

We'd allowed ourselves extra time for the journey from Snape to Leeds and we were due to arrive in Leeds city centre at 4 p.m. so we had time for sandwiches and coffee. Sitting in Luke's house, we relaxed till it was time to set off. The phone went, it was Mike.

'You are going down Roundhay Road and up the Headrow, like we said?'

'Yes. Just like we said,' I replied, my voice sharp with impatience.

'Right, well, I'm not sure but you might get a police escort into town.'

'What?'

'Yeah. I think there are some police motor-cyclists going to meet you somewhere along Roundhay Road.'

Luke, who was strapping on his helmet, stood waiting by the bike. When I told him about the police escort he looked a little incredulous. 'Yeah, right,' he muttered.

We set off slowly. Mike had said to get to Millennium Square at 4 p.m. – not earlier. The traffic was quite busy coming from the direction of Leeds and several cars blew their horns and their drivers waved encouragement at us.

As we pulled up at the Fforde Green hotel we

could see two big police bikes travelling towards us, emblazoned with blue and yellow stripes. We were stood astride our tandem waiting for the lights when they pulled alongside us, and then in front of us. Raising hands to stop the traffic, they waved us through. As we drew level with them, the leathered policeman pushed his glasses up so I could see his face.

'Take it easy now, Jane,' he said and smiled.

'Thank you,' I said, echoing Luke, and we pushed our way off as the bikes passed us to stop the traffic at the next set of lights.

Luke laughed, 'How cool is this?'

I chortled. It was such a buzz cycling into the city centre and my home town with a police escort. Passengers on buses craned their necks to see what the hold-up was. Then there was beeping of horns and waving. All the bus passengers were banging on the windows and sticking their thumbs up in encouragement as we proceeded with ease through the streets towards Leeds.

Round the roundabout by Leeds Playhouse and then up the slightly sloped Headrow in the direction of the town hall, we swung a right up towards Leeds General Infirmary and the police waved us on and sped away. We pulled on to the square in front of the white civic hall where a crowd had gathered and there were cameras and film crews waiting for us. As we arrived, the whole pack descended till we had to stop and dismount. I looked around and saw some familiar faces – friends and family – but many strangers had also turned up to see me cycle into Leeds. The cameras flashed and reporters with notebooks

89

surrounded us. I could just make out my mum's face as we were surrounded by a media pack.

We eventually arrived home. Too late to cook tea, we had a fish and chip supper. I unpacked and washed my dirty kit.

'Suzanne, have you put the laundry in the dryer?' Mike asked.

'No, I was just about to.'

Mike looked at Rebecca. 'Don't worry. I was just going to stack the dishwasher and clean the kitchen,' she said.

My head spun with the noise and normality of home after so many days of just cycling and sleep.

The following day, with all the excitement forgotten, I was once again sat in the treatment chair waiting for my chemotherapy. That evening, I prepared myself for two weeks away from home, two more weeks of cycling. I lay in bed next to Mike.

'How are you feeling?' he asked.

'I feel like I want the ride to be over. I don't even want to think about getting on the bike tomorrow.'

We set off from Rothwell Main Street outside the Yorkshire Building Society, who had helped us enormously by being our collecting point for the fundraising. With our longest day of cycling ahead of us, I had watched the weather report the night before and sighed with relief when I saw the arrows showing the wind direction as southerly – the most favourable for us on our mammoth eighty-mile leg.

The day was long. Each time my blood sugar

levels fell slightly I was overtaken by extreme nausea. Stopping and eating regularly to keep the retching to a minimum made the day draw on and on. We cycled through South Elmsall and Mexborough where the children clung to the railings of the school and cheered us as we passed. We lifted our arms and waved enthusiastically. Their rousing cheers kept us going for a couple of miles before the pit of my stomach started to rise once more.

The daylight was starting to fade as we coasted into Newark and eventually found our accommodation. Time to eat and fall straight into bed exhausted after a warming and relaxing bath.

The next day we could hear the busy A1 road as we set off from the hotel and headed off towards Melton Mowbray. We picked up some of their famous pies but Melton Mowbray seemed unwelcoming and hard to get through on the tandem. Lorry drivers seemed to be pushing close by us so we kept on cycling and stopped at the village just south of the town called Great Dalby.

As we sat on the grass, we could see the small black insects winging their way towards us attracted by our yellow cycling jackets. The sickness hadn't abated much and the effort of cycling made me retch – my head hung low, my eyes streaming for several minutes before it passed. After that I couldn't face the pork pies but managed a trusty peanut butter sandwich and a slice of malt loaf which settled my stomach.

We set off enthusiastically, heading for the village of Kibworth just off the B6047. As we turned off the main road, the small whitened farmhouses and the hedges took on a familiar feel. Although I'd not been to Kibworth for many years, it felt comfortable to be here and, turning from the village, we passed the green and went down a small road of shops to Smeeton Westerby. We stopped where the road doglegged and sat on the grass verge looking at the great gate ahead of us. I remember sitting in the minibus as a child, tired after the long journey. Dad opening the gate. Bessie the dog barking and then the sound muffled as she was shut into the stables. She was a working dog and didn't enjoy her territory being overtaken by so many strangers. Then the metal grating as the gate was pulled shut. Dad climbing back up into the minibus and driving it into the yard. Yellow straw flattened into concrete. The sweet smell of straw, the stench of sheep shit and piss, sour and strong, pervading the yard.

We tumbled out of the minibus and into the porch where a small round figure stood. 'Hello, my ducks.' My grandma greeted us and kissed each one of us as we squeezed past her and into her dining room. The table was set with heavy cutlery. Place mats showing hunting scenes were arrayed around it. The smell of fat scorched in the oven. Only a large joint cooking smells that way. The fat cooked long and hard over some hours filling the air, clinging all the way to the darkened beams above the table. The small blackened range was warm.

We padded along the tunnelled corridor, the deep-walled recess into the next room filled with spicy smells and zinging with oranges, and then into the comfortable living room with large couches. There weren't enough seats for us all and we fought over them, some of us ending up on the floor.

Luke and I looked at the gate. The white gabled end of the farmhouse has been taken back to the brickwork, herringbone patterned, it was the same but not. We peered through the gate but the yard was clean of animals. The stables where the sheep had been housed to lamb in early spring were cleaned up. The barn where the grain used to be stored was now someone's house. We walked down the lane just in front of the yard. It led to the fields we used to visit, tumbling around in the old Land Rover. Ill-fitting red wellies on our feet, we would stumble round the fields muddying ourselves. We reached the gate and rested against it. My helmet swinging from its strap at my hip, I laid my chin on to the back of my hands and looked into the field at the other side. On the left, the rough hawthorn hedge glowing green was bejewelled with tight small white and red flowers filling the air with their odd overpowering sweetness.

I stood listening but there were no lambs bleating in the field. I heard the echoes from under a small bridge of a long-past game of hide-and-seek. A golden day in a golden field at harvest time. Tumbling home in the back of a deep trailer filled with grain, watching as feet disappeared, buried under the dusty gathered crop. Desperately searching for the boot that fell from my foot as I clambered from the trailer.

Luke and I turned towards each other. 'Time to go?' I asked. He nodded, quietened, and we walked back up the small lane towards Debdale Farm and the tandem.

The sun that had bathed the farm with golden light, colouring our memories, was warm and welcoming as we arrived at Market Harborough. We cycled past the stilted black-and-white gabled grammar school. No longer a school but it's where my dad was taught. The sunshine tempted Luke and I out for a run. My legs used to the rotation of the pedals did not take easily to running and the action felt stilted and uncomfortable. The downhill stretch out of town was an effort to pump back up but we arrived back in time to wash ourselves and our clothes before Mike, Rebecca and Steven descended on us.

MIKE

Steven tugged at my left hand, ever a good yard behind so it always looked as though I was dragging him along. Morning dew was still glistening on the grass as we approached a grey-stone house on our right which had a beautiful manicured lawn the size of two tennis courts. A canopy in the centre provided shelter to some garden tables and chairs.

'Rosemary, grab the orange juice and ask Simon to help.' A middle-aged man appeared holding in both hands a tray with dishes and cutlery. He eyed Steven and me with a suspicious glance as we walked down the road.

'It's a lovely morning,' I said.

He ignored me, placing his tray on to the table.

94

He fumbled in his pocket and in an exaggerated movement he extended his arm, setting on his car alarm. Moving quicker now, indeed almost breaking into a trot, he moved to his drive entrance and shut his gate. I looked at Steven and wondered how the man could feel so threatened by us walking close to his property.

The village of Lower Slaughter was tranquil and quite magnificent. I felt inclined to write to all the Yorkshire bus companies and point out what a beautiful final destination it would be for a mystery tour. Forget Blackpool, Scarborough or Bridlington – this was the real deal, ye olde fashioned English village. The only downside to this idyllic country setting was that the locals made us feel as welcome as Boris Johnson in Liverpool. It's true that the motorhome parked so close to the village centre was the only blot on the perfect landscape but even so. As Steven and I returned to the motorhome an elderly gentleman stopped and asked us where the menu was.

'Pardon?'

'The menu.' He looked at me as though I'd spoken a different language.

Chris interjected. 'All right, mate, we're not a mobile caff – we're supporting a charity bike ride.'

'So, I can't even get a cup of tea then,' he muttered and walked off. Chris said that wasn't the first time he'd had that particular conversation.

The Cotswolds had taken me by surprise. It was quite stunning but there was just a slight air of pretentiousness about it. The beauty and tranquillity

95

of the villages was in stark contrast to the local centre, Stow-on-the-Wold, which was just one big car park even at 10.30 on a Sunday morning.

Steven, Rebecca and I joined the ride at Market Harborough with the intention of staying to the end. Suzanne had remained at home to continue studying for her imminent A levels. The prospect of a road trip had seemed exciting but as we passed through the overnight stops of Stratford, Cirencester and Wells there was an air of melancholy amongst all of us. Cabin fever had taken hold and there was a sense that we were just getting through each day as best we could. The whole point of the ride seemed to be to reach the next destination without enjoying any of the scenery and tetchiness had replaced optimism.

Psychologically the ride into Leeds had been a disaster for Jane. Seeing her family, sleeping at home and then having to set off again had been ill-conceived. The days since had been about mere survival for her – the series of long stages and the tiredness and sickness from the chemotherapy she'd received when in Leeds weighing her spirits down.

The day's ride from Cirencester to Wells had been particularly torturous; one delay after another meant a late finish. To allow Chris a day in the saddle, I'd taken the wheel of the motorhome, much to Steven's excitement. His feeling of euphoria, however, soon evaporated as he was flung from one side of the van to the other like a pea in a drum while I grappled with the controls. On the approach into Wells a white van smashed into our driver's side mirror. By the day's completion, my nerves were shredded and Steven had what appeared to be post-traumatic shock syndrome.

Pulling up at the agreed meeting point, I closed my eyes and felt the blood return back to my face. Jane was four miles further back – about twenty minutes behind.

'Is Mum here, Dad?' Steven shouted from the back.

'No, she won't be long.'

'Aawwhh.'

Although Steven had a high boredom threshold, today had proved more tedious than watching a Chris Tavare innings. Russell Fuller of Radio Five Live, who was to interview Jane when she rolled in at the end of the day, was waiting for us at the stage finish. It was unusual to meet someone whose voice was so familiar. Russell was slim and surprisingly youthful. We shook hands.

'Mike, pleased to meet you. How is Jane doing?'

'Fine. She'll be here soon. I just need to sort the kids out and park the motorhome.'

'No problem.'

I wandered back up the road as cars tore past within inches of my body. My car was already at the bed and breakfast, as we'd driven down the night before, and the Yorkshire Television crew had kindly offered to drop us back there later as we had no transport. Everything on the road seemed to be chaos – cars and bikes, equipment constantly being ferried to various locations, leapfrogging the riders throughout the southern counties. I'd never seen anyone work as hard as Martyn and Ian from Sky; riding all day, constantly looking for shots to

97

film, thinking of the scripts for the broadcasts. Then they'd unpack in the new hotel room and edit the footage until the small hours of the morning before sleeping and starting again. Every day they started the ride early, heading out up to an hour in front of Jane and Luke to buy some time at the end of the day.

As Jane and Luke bore down towards us, legs pumping in perfect symmetry, a sixty-foot juggernaut whistled past them, the draught causing the bike to lurch rightwards before spitting it out leftwards. There was a sense of vulnerability about Jane as she dismounted while Luke held the frame. Unbuckling her helmet her hair bounced back into life.

'Did you get the water?' she asked me.

'No, I couldn't find any.' As the words left my mouth I realised how lame this sounded. With her helmet clutched in the fist of her left hand, even at five foot she looked menacing. I stuttered, 'What... Well... What. We've been really busy.' I looked backwards for support, 'Haven't we been busy, Steven?'

'No, Daddy, we haven't.' My eyes bored into his forehead but he stood impassive.

'Only one thing you had to do, one measly thing and even that was too much.'

Having already destroyed the wing mirror I didn't fancy reversing the motorhome off a busy trunk road into a drive with barely a six-inch clearance at either side, so I left it to Luke and Chris. The sickening sound of metal crunching against stone vindicated my decision and I took this to be a perfect moment to beat the retreat

98

before I was dragged into an inquest.

By the time Jane had completed two television interviews, and despite the recent start of summer daylight hours, dusk was drawing in. We stopped off in Wells to find some water but this extra task merely increased Jane's irritation towards me.

Fortunately the accommodation was splendid – otherwise my coffin would have been well and truly nailed shut. By the time Jane had showered and changed hunger had overtaken us and it was nearly eight o'clock. As is usual when folks are tired, hungry and a long way from home, we became a little fractious. But because Russell was still patiently waiting for his interview we were on our best behaviour. I use that term loosely. It was turned ten o'clock before Jane had finished the interview, which was not surprisingly recorded in one take.

Next morning, Jane was already partially dressed as I awoke, her cycling undergarments providing protection from the chilly morning air.

'Come on, Mike,' she said. 'I need to eat and then be on the road.' I turned over. 'Come on.' Her voice seemed to rise an octave. A five-second rattling of the door handle preceded Steven's entry, fully dressed as if to add extra weight to Jane's words.

Three weeks cycling and Jane's midriff looked taut, her leg muscles well defined with each movement. Her face was bronzed and she was the picture of good health. We'd seen the regular TV interviews as she descended the country; her smile radiated a perfect advertisement for the outdoor life.

After six months of chemotherapy, however low in toxicity it was, she'd come alive. Yet, close up, there were the minuscule signs of weariness, her right eye not opening as far as the left, a darkness around both eyes, a sallowness of the facial features.

Jane had been up at seven; she had already sorted out her cycling kit for the day, filling water bottles and repacking her overnight bag. 'Are you going to move?' she asked. I turned over, pretending not to hear her. 'Come on, Mike, you promised you'd sort Steven out.' I heard the door close, silence in the room followed by creaks of the stairs was evidence of Jane's departure. Aware I'd gone too far I was dressed and ready in five minutes, but the damage was done and it would set a poor tone for the day.

Steven, Rebecca and I joined Chris and headed to Glastonbury for a quick visit to the Tor. Glastonbury was, as I'd imagined it would be, a refuge for those who yearned for an 'alternative' existence. I'd never seen as many dogs on strings, multicoloured wool jumpers and beards since I'd last visited Totnes. Herbal teas were the norm in the local café, the mugs were as loud as the jumpers and definitely cast at a local kiln. Many of the inhabitants looked like they'd been left behind from one of the early 1970s festivals. But it sucked you in and made you feel comfortable; the more the minutes ticked the less inclined I was to move. The peace was shattered as Steven's voice belted out, 'Get that phone, Dad!' Fifteen pairs of eyes turned and gave me a 'you're not local' look, making me feel extremely uncomfortable. Unnervingly, Steven looked at me and said, 'Well, answer it, Dad.'

It was the first of a continuous series of phone calls that kept coming throughout the next seven hours. Most of the calls were from journalists. It appeared that hostilities in Iraq would cease as the invading troops reached Baghdad, which meant that the UK media needed new stories and quickly.

So far, regular PA reports had lead to some interest in the ride but this was redundant while the news was saturated with coverage of the conflict. Little did we know how much media attention would be on Jane now that the war looked as though it was over.

JANE

We set off in good time from Launceston as we wanted an early finish and to spend some time with our families before the last day into Land's End. We could smell the salt in the air when we arrived at Wadebridge after half an hour cycling. Mike hired a bike with a tag-along, a small bike attachment that allowed Steven to cycle with him. A red flag waving at the back, Steven's little legs swung backwards and forwards as they rode along the dedicated cycle path called the Camel Trail towards Padstow.

After so many days cycling we were finally reaching the coast again after leaving it many miles back in Scotland, at Bettyhill. We stopped the bike and stood looking at the sea, lost in memories of the last few weeks. My face cracked with my widening smile as I remembered how far we had travelled. Steven and Mike pulled alongside on their hired bike.

'Have you been working hard back there?' I asked Steven. 'I couldn't see you pedalling.'

'I have, Mummy. My legs are tired now.'

I unclipped the opening of my pannier and passed him a Mars bar. He climbed from the bike and sat on a rock, his mouth soon full of chocolate.

I kissed Steven and Mike and we climbed back on the bike and set off again along the coastal road towards Newquay. Memories of the first day's cycling hugging a sea line returned as we swooped down steep winding roads.

For the last few days I'd wanted to get up and get on. I'd wished the cycling over and Land's End met. I was tired and the daily routine had taken the gloss from the adventure. It felt like a job to do. A job to finish. Now here we were at our last stopping point before Land's End. I was relieved and could look forward to the last day on the bike.

The small town sat on a cliff top and the wind blew as Luke and I sat looking out to sea. A little way down the hill there was a sandy beach and a small pub. We were dressed and ready early for our final day. A last fifty miles to cycle. We were heading away from the north Cornish coast down to Penzance on the southern seaboard and then to Land's End. I could taste the cream tea that had been calling to me all the way through Devon and on into Cornwall. No visit to the west country could be complete without one. We arranged to meet Mike in Marazion at lunchtime.

'Foot up,' Luke called. I raised my left foot and rested it on the pedal. We pushed down and set off. When we had started in Scotland we'd been blessed with fair weather, but it was hard to imagine spring. As we had cycled down the country it was as if spring had burst upon us. Golden daffodils in Leeds. Lambs in Leicestershire. Here the daffodils drooped and the tulips had tight buds waiting to show their colours. Here, the little lambs of Leicestershire were now bounding, bouncing creatures as we cycled on towards Land's End.

We could see the castled hill with the National Trust-run priory buildings as we dropped into Marazion. We spotted the gardens climb up out of the sea above the rocks to meet the walls of the castle. St Michael's Mount causeway was open and people were walking out to the small island across it before it was cut off by the tide.

We ate Cornish pasties sat on the benches by the sea, the hot potato burning my mouth and the wind catching Rebecca's hair. She held it back with one hand while she ate. Mike looked anxiously at his watch.

'You'd better get going,' he said. Luke rolled his eyes and I shrugged my shoulders at him.

'We'll finish our lunch first, if that's okay,' I muttered as I took another mouthful. 'Don't forget you promised me a cream tea today when we finish.' I threw the debris in the bin and Luke wheeled the bike out on to the road ready to set off.

'See you later.' Mike came and caught me, kissed me on the cheek. 'You're nearly there, fantastic job, the both of you. See you at the finish.'

We set off towards Penzance our legs moving smoothly, the excitement of the finish making the bike ride and our pedalling swift. Fifteen minutes later the bike groaning, our legs aching, our backs bent low we pushed and pushed up the cruel hill that seemed to climb straight up and out of Penzance. Cars overtook us, forcing us to slow and drawing a curse from my lips.

We stood at the top, recovered ourselves before we pushed on, eager to finish. The road curled through the countryside, high hedgerows on either side of us, small tracks to the left and right. We were so close now. Each signpost counted down the miles to Land's End. We could make out the sea to the left of us as we crested hills and then we were left in the countryside as we rolled down into small vales. At last we came to the signpost. Left to Land's End or right to Penzance.

'Which way?' Luke asked. 'Are you ready for this?'

'Absolutely.'

'They should have a brass band or something playing,' said Luke as our legs circled and we headed towards the low dull buildings that made up the finish of Land's End.

'What's that?' Luke asked. We could make out a few people and I could see a white line across the road. We passed smoothly across the black tarmac.

'This is it,' I said. 'We've finished.'

Our front wheel crossed the white line that

showed the end of the ride, and behind my dark glasses tears filled my eyes. A camera pointed at us as we stood at the end of our long journey. Luke's face creased with emotion, his eyes glazed. The journey had been made up of so many emotions – eagerness to cycle and enjoy the trip and then eagerness just to be finished. Then sadness that the cycling would be over. At times, the days on the bike had felt like work, another day just to get through. At other times, though, it had felt like a huge adventure. Now it was over and we would be home in a few days' time.

'I don't think I want to cycle for a few days' now.'

'Too right,' Luke replied.

CHAPTER 3

April 2003

MIKE

Which wazzock had suggested that we all run the marathon after Jane finished the ride? After her finish yesterday, we could have celebrated, got drunk, gone home to a welcoming bed and familiar surroundings. Instead, last night's celebrations had finished by 10 p.m., although my head was testament that even that was too late.

Eleven hours later we were walking across Blackheath towards the starting line. We'd scrounged a lift from a *Sky News* crew and as a consequence were unfashionably early. The common was littered with pockets of runners heading across it as if following a siren's call. We ambled very slowly towards the start.

I reflected how a year ago we'd been in the same situation with Jane being interviewed by the BBC just before her first marathon. What a difference a year had made. Although, of course, we still talked about Jane's health – the cancer and the treatments – our discussions of these subjects were now overshadowed by conversations about Jane's future. People no longer asked, 'What's the prognosis?'; it seemed a redundant thing to ask. Instead, it was: 'What's Jane up to next?' or 'How's Jane's training going?'

Sometimes, it was possible to forget Jane was ill at all – the times when we were all concentrating normally on the present and the immediate future plans.

As the hooter for the start sounded, Jane and I didn't budge from our seated position on the grass. There was no point. We waited an extra five minutes as most athletes crossed and then made our way to the crowds of runners. I was determined not to run an inch longer than the 26 miles 385 yards.

'Why are we here Mike?' Jane asked.

'Beats me.'

As I approached the Isle of Dogs the course took me right past our hotel. The urge to stop, enter, shower, change and go to bed was overwhelming. I pictured Jane miles ahead and it was only because of the absolute piss-take I'd be subjected to by everyone that I carried on.

With some relief I managed to run/walk the last few miles and reached the Mall after five hours forty minutes. Pathetic. The only salvation was that Jane was behind me, quite how I couldn't imagine.

JANE

'How are you?' asked Dr Velikova. 'I see you finished your bike ride, and then you ran the marathon.'

'Well, I'd hardly call it running,' I replied. 'It was a long day and I can officially say cycling doesn't make you running fit.'

'Were there any problems?' she asked, flicking the curl of hair from her eyes as she looked at me.

'No,' I laughed. 'I think I had less problems than anyone else. I am still a bit saddle sore but I'm fine.'

Dr Velikova scanned my notes. 'Well, as far as treatment goes, you've had about as much Vinorelbine as we would like to give you. We'll carry on with the Herceptin and I think we should maybe try one of the hormonal therapies again, but not Tomoxifen.'

'You mean no more chemo?' I asked, surprised.

'Yes. We sometimes give it a little longer, but we should finish now.' I sat up at that news. What a relief. My back straightened and my shoulders relaxed. I'd been having chemo for so long I couldn't imagine what the week would be like

107

without the tiredness and nausea. 'Also,' she continued. 'You might like to think about having Herceptin every three weeks instead of weekly.'

'That would be great,' I said. The thought of not being tied to the hospital once a week was wonderful. It was hard to think how much freedom it would allow me.

Walking from the hospital with Mike back to the car, my step was light. I had been dreading another four weeks of chemo and now I didn't need to any longer.

'You'll be able to start training for the triathlons,' Mike said.

'I think I'll give myself a couple of weeks off before that.'

'You need to start going to the pool. Get yourself fit for the swimming.'

I raised my eyebrows and scowled at Mike's back as he stepped out into the road.

The following Monday the sun spread from the side of the curtains. Turning over in bed I huddled under the covers a little further. My foot stretched out hitting a cold spot in the sheets, and I withdrew it, curling myself up to enjoy the warmth as the covers hugged my body and I dozed back to sleep. I felt Mike turn towards me and his arm lay heavily over my shoulder. It seemed oddly indulgent and such a long time since we just lay in bed with no need to rush off to work or for me to climb out of bed and into cycling shorts.

The door squeaked and opened slowly, Steven stood in the shadows, his white comfort-nappy drooping on to the floor.

'Is it up time yet?' he asked.

'Nearly,' I said. 'Come and get a cuddle.' I shuffled towards the middle of the bed ignoring Mike's protests, nudging him to make him move.

The letterbox clattered and the post thudded on to the floor.

'The postman's been,' Steven said as he pulled the covers back and slid to the floor. 'Shall I get the letters, Mummy?'

'Go on, then.' I heard him skipping down the steps one at a time, picking up the post and then returning to the bedroom.

'Yours, yours, yours, yours. Oh, no, the visa bill.' Mike handed over a wad of post. 'Open this one first.'

I took the white heavily embossed envelope from him. The words 'Downing Street' were stamped on the front. 'That'll be your knighthood, Sir Jane,' he said. I opened the envelope and read the letter asking me to accept an inclusion in the Queen's Birthday Honours.

'Do you think I ought to accept it?' I asked Mike as I passed him the letter.

'Yes, of course.'

'I don't know why they're bothering honouring me,' I said.

'What? After all you've done, of course you deserve it.'

MIKE

After the high of finishing the ride, the return to

109

humdrum routine sent us all into a downward spiral. The planning had taken up much of the last six months and the anticipation of the event had lightened up an otherwise gloomy winter. The fundraising had been fantastically successful, like a downhill snowball gathering momentum, so the £100,000 target was easily achieved. Many media and commercial requests, shop openings, charity functions and speaking engagements for Jane flooded in, mainly from those who'd shown no interest until the successful completion. Jane, though, had no appetite for any of it, so we went into hibernation – only fulfilling engagements we had agreed to prior to the ride.

But now it was all over, there was a void in our lives. Like students finishing exams we found ourselves with an abundance of time but no focus. At home we'd all become a little independent of Jane so there was a readjustment to be done too.

Weekends weighed heavily on us; when you've not had a free one for months to now have six on the bounce seemed to create its own pressure. Suzanne's A levels were due to commence and in truth it would be a bloody relief when she went to university. At seventeen, she had been trying to push the boundaries of her independence for some months and the living room had become a minefield of barbed comments and teenage sulks; and I wasn't the only culprit. I'm convinced that there's a part of every teenage girl's brain that forces her to behave in an utterly unpleasant manner to anyone who lives with her and behave impeccably with anyone else.

To make matters worse, as Suzanne was probably leaving this phase, Rebecca was just starting to enter it. On some occasions, it seemed that there was a magnetic force between both girls where they would take turns at being unpleasant. One's pleasantness would feed the mood of the other's tantrums, and they would swap roles with consummate ease and efficiency.

It was therefore with some relief that we liberated ourselves from the teenage angst and escaped on a Saturday morning to enter a traffic jam to Ilkley. Jane had a fanciful notion that we could become a family for whom cycling became the hobby of choice. The central component of this would be to buy a tandem on which Steven could ride stoker. Swept along on a tide of enthusiasm I'd agreed to have a look at the options. As a notion I supported it, the major obstacle for me was the thought of exercise being the central weekend theme, especially on two wafer-thin wheels. I was conscious of the recent TV pictures of me cycling, images which had generated an inordinate amount of unwarranted piss-taking and wry smiles from mild acquaintances. There wasn't, as I saw it, any need to perpetuate this contempt.

The bike shop was tucked away in an attractive courtyard of garages within spitting distance of the town centre. Their selection of bikes catered for the mountain bike enthusiast, but they also had a good selection of tandems; an item they said was selling three times more than in other years. Steven and I trailed Jane as if on an invisible lead as she looked at a variety of alternatives, all of which seemed unsuitable for Steven. It seemed

111

as though he was at a crossover age – too big for those bikes where he'd just be a passenger but too small for a proper tandem.

Jane looked at a yellow tandem then at Steven. 'Will you sit on it, Steven, please.' Steven sat on the stoker position while the shop assistant propped the bike.

'It's too big,' he said, trying to make his legs stretch to the pedals.

'There's nothing we can do here. We can't shorten the shaft as there's not enough space and the seat is in its lowest position,' the assistant said. Jane looked at Steven, clearly trying to work out how many inches he'd have to grow before he could use it.

'It's seven hundred pounds, Mike, and it'll be some time before he gets any use out of it.' The crucial part of the sentence remained unsaid.

Jane looked at me and it brought home that all purchases were temporary and that only instant gratification was relevant to Jane. How often people of an older generation had said to her, 'Oh, well, it will see my days out'; a comment always likely to infuriate someone whose days were going to fall decades short of the orator. Anticipation of future pleasure was irrelevant; we needed good times and we needed them now. Even so, it became apparent that Jane's plan would be frustrated.

'I'm just going to get some spares for my bike,' Jane said. 'I won't be more than five minutes.' This was Jane's polite attempt at telling us to bugger off and leave her in peace. Steven looked at a photograph of Lance Armstrong while I perused a collection of leaflets. Most were small flyers advertising local charity rides or outings of interest. One with quite an unattractive photo – but is there any other – of the Millennium Dome caught my eye. It was entitled 'Rome to the Dome'. I looked across at Jane who was still examining cycling gloves.

Since coming back from London I'd been looking at options for another fundraising opportunity. More often than not, Jane had frozen me out before I'd even got halfway through the first sentence but, recently, I'd sensed a thawing; not much of one admittedly but at least something to work on. I knew I could succeed with persistence.

Rome seemed perfect, Jane loved Italy and France, and she's Catholic. I scanned the blurb and was surprised to note that the ride's distance was quite paltry and it wasn't much of a challenge, as it avoided any serious climbs and took a very direct route. This was worth thinking about, especially as a major constraint was the need to do an event in the European Union where Jane would have free health insurance.

From a fundraising perspective it ticked a lot of boxes. It certainly impressed me that someone should cycle from Rome to London. And if someone like Jane were to do it, well, it would take people's breath away. I folded the leaflet carefully and placed it in my back pocket.

'What's that, Dad?'

'It's Mum's next cycle ride, though she doesn't know it yet. It's a secret so don't tell her, will you?'

'How'd the exam go?' Jane asked Suzanne later

that evening.

'Fine.' Suzanne moved her fork scooping up an unfeasibly large mound of mash potatoes.

'Are you going to see Granddad?' Rebecca asked me. 'Can I come?'

'Me too,' said Steven.

'Rebecca can. It's too late for you, Steven.' Jane was vehemently shaking her head indicating, although I was already aware, that it wouldn't be appropriate.

'I'd love to but can't really,' Suzanne added.

'Don't worry. Granddad wouldn't have approved of skipping revision to see him. Anyway, you can keep an eye on Steven while mum goes for a cycle.'

'What?' Jane looked incredulous.

'Well you've got a half ironman looming.'

'It's three months away and I'm cycle fit.'

'Is that what you call it?'

'You cheeky sod.'

'Anyway, it'll be good practice for next year's marathon tandem ride.'

'Mum!' Rebecca piped up. 'Fantastic, where are you going?'

'He's kidding.'

'I thought Paris or Berlin to Leeds,' I said. 'Can I leave the table?'

'You can't take it with you.' They all shouted the latest recitation of our family joke.

JANE

Slumped in a plastic chair at the Leeds Inter-

114

national Swimming Pool, I placed my head on the bag on the table and closed my eyes. Opening them a few seconds later, I checked the clock at the back of the staff area. It was still only 7.10 in the morning.

It was a tiring training regime, but I couldn't help feeling a certain smugness in having managed to fit in some swimming before work. It meant I would be able to tick off the first part of another day's training. A 1500 metre swim before work, and a 5 kilometre run or a 15 mile bike ride in the evening. I had to fit in my training as best as I could round work and family. It was a challenge but it was just about manageable.

In the evening Steven went to a friend's birthday party straight from school, which meant I was able to have a short rest before my hour's cycle ride.

I yawned as I rose from my bed, groggy from the small nap but keen to make the most of the time I had left that evening. Lifting the bike from the garage, I shut the door and cursed having forgotten my helmet. I pushed the door up and open and retrieved it and then locked the garage.

It was a hot day and the yellow jacket clung as sweat poured from me. I pedalled slowly down through Rothwell and through the traffic lights and enjoyed the cool air stripping past me as I headed for the small curved bridge out of the town. It was a tight walled bend, and I looked behind me as I pedalled through, making sure there were no cars that would catch me unawares. After the bridge I pushed down a little harder and carried on down the road – redbrick terraces on my left, fields on my right. A car came alongside me and then slowed down to my pace. I resisted looking into it; I got enough unprovoked abuse from motorists without attracting any more attention.

I could hear loud music and young men's voices from inside the car and tried to ignore their comments.

'Look at that!' one spat.

'Bloody cyclists. I hate them,' said another.

A hand appeared from the front passenger window. I was a little unnerved by now. The hand receded a little and then pushed forward, digging into my side with a brutal force as the car sped off. My bike fell to the side of the road, and I went with it. With my ankle caught between the kerb and the bike, I collided sharply with the corner of a terraced house. I jolted my shoulder against the brickwork on my way down to the ground and I lay momentarily shaken as the car stopped about fifty yards in front of me. Pulling myself from under the bike, I stepped into the road. The car reversed a little towards me – I could still hear the laughter and abuse from inside.

Once the young lads had watched my discomfort, they sped off laughing but not before I'd taken down the registration number, make and colour of the car, scribbling them on a scrap of paper in my saddlebag as I sat quaking on the kerb distraught by what had just happened.

My face was tear-stained, my left leg raw and dripping with blood when the police arrived a little while later. Some people who had witnessed the assault had stopped to check I was okay.

They'd been shocked at the cold-blooded nature of the push.

I was angry by the time the police arrived. 'They didn't care if they hurt me,' I told them tearfully. 'They even stopped to make sure they had hurt me; I could hear them laughing at me.'

'You need to go to casualty to have your injuries checked,' the policeman said.

I nodded.

'Do you need some help to get home?'

'No, it's not far. I'll cycle back, thanks,' I replied.

His eyes opened a little wider. 'Are you sure?' he asked. 'You don't really look fit to cycle.'

'No honestly. I'm fine.' Still, my leg was sore and the gash at my ankle opened again as I hauled myself on to the bike and set off, pushing my bruised body home.

That night in bed, I slowly peeled away the sheets that had stuck to my leg. The pain made me gasp; it felt like I was ripping off huge dressings from the scrapes all down my left leg. Road rash is the cyclists' term for when you rub your skin off on the road in a collision. I had had my road rash scrubbed clean of debris at St James's casualty department. The nurse had carefully scrubbed away at the wound with a toothbrush and cleaning solution.

Thanks to the registration number, the police found the car and took someone in for questioning. But I couldn't identify them and I couldn't place them at the scene. So all they could do was interview the lads who owned the car about the event. Still, I hoped that they got a good talking

117

to. I wanted to shake them, scare them as much as they had scared me.

It took weeks for my leg to heal. All the swimming I had pushed myself to do, all the fitness I had built up was now lost as I couldn't start training properly again until the wounds had closed.

I continued to cycle but my confidence was low. One afternoon, cycling through the lanes not far from home I could hear a car coming up behind me, loud music blaring. Shaking, I stopped and pulled the bike from the road, watching the car speed past.

White faces peered at me from the windows as they raced past and for minutes afterwards all I could do was sit on the roadside, calming myself, as I was too frightened to set off. My legs and hands trembled, my face flushed with fear. Another car and then another car passed, my stomach muscles loosened and I wiped my mouth, rinsing it with water to take away the dryness. The experience just weeks before had left my confidence in tatters, but eventually I gathered myself and slowly cycled the five miles home.

MIKE

Our coach, third in a convoy of six, pulled into the large windswept car park in Filey, North Yorkshire. It was a grey stretch of land, sparsely populated with dogs and their owners having their morning walk. I had packed away Steven's travel chess and asked him to put on his jumper, coat and hat – looking out at the weather it was

118

clear factor thirty wouldn't be required today.

Outside, coachloads of children began to disembark. It could have been any deserted car park in the country. It seemed a little uninspired to have the annual school trip to the same place every year; this was the third time we'd visited. But that said, the only thing curbing the kids' enthusiasm was the low cloud, single digit temperature and drizzle.

'Can we go to craaazzzy golf, Dad?' Steven asked.

'Definitely, in a little while,' I said and he ran off to talk to two of his friends, his Toy Story rucksack swinging from his back.

I felt a burst of fatherly pride. The location or weather was suddenly irrelevant. This was a precious day; one for father and son. If there was such a thing as a silver lining to Jane's illness, it was the chance I'd got to take on a more direct parenting role. School trips, dental appointments, clubs and activities were my primary responsibility. Jane had, over the years, taken the lion's share of the household chores – she was the engine room of the house. Her continuing ill health, though, had ensured that I shouldered more than I would have done in normal circumstances. And it was essential I took on the tasks such as dental checkups – after all, when Jane was gone, there would be no one else to make sure the kids went.

But the truth was, I loved it; well, maybe not the housework, but certainly the parenting. Caught in the need to develop a career, there is a tendency to miss the children growing up; not being able to attend sports days or nativity plays.

Now there was a greater sense of not wanting to miss out on their development, an acknowledgement that time is precious, that these years of their lives wouldn't be repeated. Because of the age gaps it was already apparent that Suzanne and Rebecca were moving on with their lives and our role as guiding figures was disappearing.

'Steven!' I shouted.

'What, Dad?' He ran back to join me, looking up expectantly. Like a fussy mother I took off his grey fleeced hat. It was shaped in the style of a First World War flying helmet with flaps covering his ears. It was not something seen often and despite all the times he left it at school or lost it, it returned unscathed.

'Let's go down the cliff path to see if we can find the sea.'

'Okay.'

We descended rapidly to the beach which looked like a mile-long strip of mud; some kids already playing half-naked had it stuck to them like mud-wrestlers. I find the sea invigorating, life affirming; there's something that reinforces the view that no matter what life will continue and that individually we are so unimportant. I've never needed counselling or help to make sense of our situation but occasionally it was crucial to remember how insignificant I am and put some context to life. Watching Steven run ahead, the sea cast a long landscape with only a solitary tanker moving across the horizon.

By eleven thirty, out of sheer boredom we decided to have lunch. We'd had a game of putting, half price because the attendant was 'ashamed at the state of green' and I didn't argue as indeed it looked like it doubled as part of a motocross circuit.

We'd visited the lifeboat station and the boat-less boating lake before. Filey hadn't changed in the last twelve months.

I decided we should head off for a walk. Climbing out of town we met a group of children and parents.

'Hi, Steve,' they chorused.

'Hi ya,' he replied as we passed them.

The parents whom I knew from the kids' parties and the like stopped to ask how the day was going.

'Slowly,' I said.

'How's Jane?' one of the mums asked. Young and slim she seemed to be from a generation younger than myself.

'She's fine, thank you,' I heard myself saying. I'd figured a long time ago that no one actually wants to know the truth as it's quite difficult to listen to and can come across as whingeing.

'Has she recovered from the assault?'

The question knocked me off guard. We'd been meticulous at ensuring that as few people knew of it as possible as we didn't want it reaching the press for fear of provoking further attacks. Sensing my surprise she continued, 'I was driving behind Jane.'

Jane had mentioned that there'd been another parent from school behind who'd kindly stopped to help, but she'd not known her.

'Her legs are quite badly marked, but the physical scars will heal quicker than the psychological one.'

'She was lucky. I was quite a long way behind and only saw how high the bike went up in the air and how hard Jane hit the wall. When she was just lying there I thought she must be very badly injured. They could have killed her.'

'I know. We realise she's been lucky in a perverse sense. Thanks for speaking to the police and helping them find the water bottle they were drinking from.'

'When are they due in court?'

'They're not.' I shook my head. 'There's a mixture of DNA in the bottle as they shared it. Although they know who the lads are, the police can't say who was sitting where in the car. They need to identify the driver and who threw the punch.'

She stared at me incredulous. 'That's ridiculous. They should be able to charge all of them.'

'I know. It's bloody frustrating. The car was what they call a pool car, shared by a number of people, used for minor criminal activity, no tax, no insurance et cetera. They'd caused quite a bit of devastation that afternoon but nothing can be proved. The same lads are also known for taking photographs of police officers as they come off duty as a kind of intimidation, so there was a desire to get them to court.'

'Did they question them?'

'Yes, they've done all they can. When they picked up one of the lads, he said, "Is this about the cyclist?" but that proved nothing.'

She shook her head. 'It's all wrong,' she sighed.

'I agree. Jane's a bit more pragmatic than me,

I'd have wanted them stringing up.'

'Did they know it was Jane?'

'No, that would have made it a lot more serious. I've been given the name and address of the person responsible but I don't think retribution would help, apart from making me feel better in the short term.' Steven had come back to join us and was shuffling from side to side, as always he was being patient but he was becoming noticeably cold. 'Anyway,' I said, keen to move on. 'Thanks for all your help.'

As I trudged off I reflected on the incident. We knew that, as a lone woman cyclist often tens of miles from home on deserted country lanes, Jane was vulnerable. We were well versed on the risks of punctures, accidents or ill health. But at no time had vicious assaults even entered our imagination. But it made us think. We'd received various hate mail letters, usually from people not believing Jane was poorly or containing abuse at the so-called neglect of the kids. We'd even received one letter from the head of a cancer support group complaining that it made her breast cancer patients feel inadequate.

As a result Jane and I had questioned whether to continue with the charitable work. It was of no personal benefit to us, indeed perversely there was every chance that the very people who perpetrated such hatred for Jane had a friend or relative who was benefiting from the money Jane had raised. Why, we wondered sometimes, should we give a toss? Jane was going to die whatever we did.

But despite our reservations, we figured our initial reasons for raising money had not changed.

It's important to see the goodness in society and not concentrate on negative elements.

By 2.30 p.m., with no improvement in the inclement weather and the limited attractions of Filey exhausted, we were ready to go home. But noticing a quiet public house, Steven and I entered and I bought a pint, a coke and two packets of crisps. Out came the travel chess, and on the pub television we copped a clear view of a sun-drenched Wimbledon. We enjoyed a pleasant, and warm, thirty minutes, diving below the frosted glass of the pub window every time someone from Steven's school passed by outside. It's amazing how old skills return.

The enclosed patient garden of Ward 24 was a tranquil oasis inside the busy Airedale Hospital. It was midsummer and, despite the cloudy day, you didn't need a jacket to keep warm, even at 6.30 p.m. Walking in circles aimlessly, I had the mobile pressed to my ear. On the third ring, Jane answered. 'Hi, Mike, how's your dad?'
    'He died, ten minutes ago.'
    'Oh, I'm so sorry. How's your mum?'
    I paced around, avoiding the urge to cry, desperately fighting back the tears, 'She's fine; they've just gone to get a doctor. It was very peaceful. I'm going to hang on here for another hour or so then I'll head home.'
    'There's no rush. Be with your mum as long as necessary.'
    'Thanks, love. See you.'
    I slipped the phone back into my jeans pocket

and wept silently for a few seconds before regaining my composure. It had been a real privilege to share the last few hours of my dad's life in a serene environment with my mum, his sister Joyce and her husband Robert.

My mum had played Johnny Cash intermittently on a portable cassette player she'd brought with her and the whole experience had been much better than I could have imagined. In twelve hours' time we were due to go on our annual family holiday to Alès in the South of France, miles from normal tourist areas as it was the only villa available. We were aware that my dad's death was imminent and would inevitably happen just before we went to France or while we were away. Jane, Rebecca, Suzanne and Steven had said their goodbyes the previous Saturday, but I'd visited daily since.

It was a dilemma as to whether to proceed with our holiday plans. I was acutely aware that quality family time with Jane was so precious – was this our last summer holiday? As usual, Jane's only concerns were for others – in this case Mum and myself. In truth I couldn't have even considered going while my dad was still alive. Mum had already agreed to hold the funeral over for three weeks until we returned and I know what my dad would have said about it.

It's a rare thing nowadays for anyone to be able to take time out to meditate and with our particularly hectic schedule it was almost impossible. Yet during my dad's final hours, I found a more substantive peace than I'd experienced before while going to mass once a week. It was a time to reflect on his life, his relationship with me, our similarities and influence.

Before the last few days of his life, I was unsure how I'd cope having to watch someone die. Now I knew I'd manage.

CHAPTER 4

July 2003

JANE

The last road up from Nîmes towards Alès was long and tiresome. Cars dawdled and the road was too busy and too narrow to allow us to overtake, so it was a relief when we finally turned off at our destination of Vezenobres. We found the narrow road that led towards our holiday cottage and turned down it, looking for the next sign.

Pulling up outside the cottage set back from the road behind a high fence, we looked for a way to open the gate, which was locked. An Alsatian dog in the house opposite took a great deal of interest in us, so I remained in the car away from its great yawning mouth full of teeth. It nosed round us while we waited for someone to come.

Finally, a small round woman, her face creased from years in the sun, stumbled across from the dog's house and, flourishing a key, opened up the gate and gave us a tour of the house. Her English was poor, as was our secondary school French, so communication was difficult.

The inside of the villa was dimly lit. The kitchen was small and it looked like it hadn't been updated since the 1950s. The furniture was bulky and dark, the dusty sideboard like a large black coffin. The whole house had an eerie feel. The villa had the use of a pool, which we'd all been excited about. The only problem was that it was guarded by the unfriendly Alsatian. When I realised this, my already fraught nerves from the journey and the long week before nearly snapped.

We dragged our suitcases and the box of food from the car and settled in. The small gite was so depressing. So much so that rather than spend time in it, it forced us to take more days out. Mike had set his heart on driving to Mont Ventoux, one of the Haute category climbs of the Tour de France, to see it for himself for the first time.

We set off to drive through the Grand Canyon du Verdon and then up the climb to the top of Mont Ventoux. As we entered the gorge, we could see the road on the other side cutting across the front of the dizzying drop.

'Wow, look at that,' Mike said as he pulling into a viewing place. Cyclists crept slowly along, like bright jewels stringing the road. Suzanne clutched the seat as we looked down at the gorge below, a tiny glint from the small stream so far beneath us.

'I'd love to cycle through here,' I said. 'Everything is just so enormous, incomprehensible.'

'It's just beautiful,' Mike said in agreement.

'Do you have to drive so close to the edge?' said

127

Suzanne, as she turned her head dramatically away from the drop.

We circled round the gorge, following the meandering course of the canyon that towered up to 700 metres. Whichever part you were in, it couldn't hide the scale of the ravine. We stopped the car, got out and stood looking across its length. I peered down to the bottom and slowly brought my eyes up to the top of the mountain, trying to take the view in. The green and brown against light limestone, the white sheer cliffside looming up and up and up to meet the harsh blue sky.

It was a long drive towards Mont Ventoux. The road took many winding turns till we drew close to Sault. We followed the line of cars grinding their way uphill in low gear, pausing to slowly overtake cyclists who were steadily climbing this beast as if on some pilgrimage. I swivelled in my seat and glimpsed the dusty face of one cyclist, whose cheeks were pink and gleaming through the sweat rivulets. His eyes were set dead straight ahead, his head hung low, mouth open and moving as if in a silent prayer, as he coaxed himself up past dozens of painted names of famous cyclists who had passed this way before.

Further on, we passed other cyclists who had dismounted from their bikes and who stood looking at the Tommy Simpson Memorial that was littered with the debris of water bottles and coloured cycling caps. Tommy Simpson was the British cyclist who died on Mont Ventoux during the 1967 Tour de France. The memorial looked like a white angel as we passed by, slowing down to look through the windows.

Mike pointed out the steady progression of cyclists as they paused at the top.

'Just think, if this ride comes off that'll be you next year,' he said. I laughed, having hobbled painfully up here from the car.

'How am I going to be able to cycle up that?' I leant over, peering down. 'You could barely drive up it.'

'That's what'll be so fantastic, and that's what training's for,' he replied. I smiled at him, wondering what other mad ideas he might have for me.

'I'm serious,' he said. 'It'll be fantastic. Just think what it will be like to get up here on a bike.'

'Yeah, Mum, that sense of achievement,' Suzanne joined in.

'You can butt out,' I said before they got too carried away.

Yet I regretted not having my bike with me. My legs itched to be cycling and I was ready to go home and start some serious training.

MIKE

Jane was distracted, staring down into her lap as if contemplating an invisible newspaper crossword. Our holiday mood was overshadowed by an unspoken gloomy force, whether it had been Dad's death, the bloodthirsty Alsatian next door or the unbearable, unseasonable heat it had not been idyllic. In Jane's circumstances life is lived with an acute desire for perfection; this is especially so while on holiday. For me it manifests in a desire to fill each day with activity, a desire to engineer fun; a policy destined for failure.

There seemed to be a desire among all of us to be at home, the knowledge we were holidaying on false pretences. The trip to Mont Ventoux had ignited Jane's enthusiasm for a continental cycling adventure. Over the next few days, our conversations were increasingly about how and when we'd do it, not if.

Jane grabbed a bottle of water from the car and began to stretch her legs. The car's temperature gauge had read 17 degrees when we'd set off from the holiday home at eight thirty. Now, ninety minutes later on the beach front of La Grande Motte, it had reached 28 degrees. Both Rebecca and Jane were fully kitted out for their training run; Suzanne meanwhile had only a suntan on her mind.

'When are you going to do some training, Suzanne?' I asked.

'Eventually, maybe tomorrow.' Suzanne discarded her T-shirt into the car boot.

'Yes, of course you are, Suzanne,' Rebecca said.

'Whatever.'

'It's only three weeks to the London Triathlon and you've not done a scrap of training,' Rebecca said.

'I'll still beat you.'

'Yeah, course you will, glory girl,' Rebecca said as she swapped her running shirt for the third time.

Jane, whose patience was beginning to wear thin, stood waiting to set off. 'Come on, Becca, before it gets too hot,' she said, placing her running eyewear on her head.

I shrugged at Jane. 'How far are you going?'

'Don't know. It depends how I feel. I'll do thirty minutes with Becca to start with.'

Beads of sweat were forming on my brow and we had only been standing in the car park for five minutes. Rebecca and Jane set off slowly, Jane struggling not to race ahead and keep in line with Becca's laconic, lazy running style.

An hour later I noticed Jane stretching and cooling off against a slated wooden fence surrounding a beach front restaurant. She swatted the air around her, a cloud of flies were circulating about the waste bins nearby. I winced as I watched her leg reach for the top of the fence, far higher than looks comfortable for anyone older than eight. The knowledge that her bone could just snap – a symptom of her disease – sent a shiver down my spine.

She hadn't noticed me looking at her, and wandering back to join us she had the smug smile of someone who'd exercised and who was just about to preach to a congregation of the lazy. This particular indolent soul was just taking a monster bite from a monster doughnut, which instantly lost its appeal as she sauntered over.

'Did you have a good run?' I asked, there was hardly a drop of perspiration on her and she looked sickeningly healthy.

After seventeen days away, we arrived back home on the Sunday and dad's funeral was arranged for the Tuesday in Settle. My dad had lived there all his seventy-four years. The elderly lady two doors away remembered him being born; the funeral director Duncan had been in the year above me at infant and secondary school. It's that kind of town.

My extended family had not gathered in Settle since my sister's wedding some sixteen years earlier and it was strange to see so many relatives back here; if only the circumstances were different.

Because the church was only a few hundred yards from my mum's, I'd intended to walk there, but she insisted I sat in the car. Duncan set off on foot with the cortege following him and that's when I could see why Mum had put her foot down. It felt very proper and totally appropriate. With supreme dignity, Duncan stopped the market day traffic so that the cortege could make its slow progress.

I recalled images of my dad: handsomely beating the other dads on school sports days; the fire alarm sounding in Settle, then watching for my dad to go running or biking to the station, or for the engine to appear; and latterly walking out for a pint with him on a Sunday night.

There is so much rushing about in life that even the simplest things can be undervalued. Each day I looked at Jane and discovered something new. At times I stared at her, wanting to savour every last memory. She'd say, 'What are you looking at?' and I'd reply, 'Not much.' Our family had come to treat as precious everyday events. We'd managed to slow down life, and heighten our senses when it came to what most people regard as the mundane because we knew that some day

Jane would not be around to enjoy them.

The church was packed. A funeral makes you reassess how transient life is. Things that you get heated up about are, in truth, not worth worrying about. Had I achieved anything by going to Manchester to study law? Or permitting the bank to move me around on a whim? My dad's life had been straightforward and he'd thoroughly enjoyed it; he'd been to two Olympics and even seen England win the World Cup. I looked around the full church, at all the people who had come to pay their last respects to my father, and suspected his life had been substantially enriched by living in a small community. Should I get to be his age and live in the city, I wondered who I would know. Who would be at my funeral? I thought how perverse it was that the more people you live amongst, the fewer you know.

Jane and I had always harboured ambitions of leaving Leeds and moving to the dales, Langcliffe or Stainforth, but these hopes had been dashed with the diagnosis as we needed to be near her hospital care.

Not long after my dad's funeral I went with Jane to meet Mark Hayward from a PR company called 1090. They were organising the publicity for the Sherborne Half Ironman and wanted Jane's commitment to the event. Of all the events Jane did in 2002, the London Triathlon was the most successful for catching people's imagination – especially those from a sporting background. The triathlon had benefited from coverage in both the Sydney Olympics and Manchester's Commonwealth Games and its star was ascending, especially for runners looking for a different type of challenge. As a multidisciplinary event, it was more rewarding than the drag of long runs.

For lay observers it seems like a sport for fitness-obsessed athletes so when Jane competed in it, it made people realise that what she was achieving was quite extraordinary.

Last year's major achievement, the London Triathlon, was this year's training run for the half ironman. Both Suzanne and Becca had agreed to take part to help boost the fundraising as it was a new angle to reach the media. More importantly, it created a unique family weekend.

Despite Suzanne's reluctance to be in the media spotlight she'd agreed to do interviews, so on Saturday dinner-time the three of them were sitting on a pontoon being interviewed for the BBC. An aqua-blue cloudless sky provided a perfect backdrop, together with the new apartments on the South Bank. A series of dock cranes stood to attention, yellow race markers bobbed in the unattractive sludge masquerading as water. Jane sat alongside Suzanne, Rebecca behind like a rear passenger looking through the front seats. I'd chastised Jane for agreeing to be interviewed on the pontoon as I knew the slight rocking on the water could adversely affect her balance for months. I'd long since known that the more I objected the less effect my words would have so I'd not pushed it, but just sat with a disgruntled look on my face tutting and rolling my eyes. All three looked in perfect health, a wonderful mother and daughters' moment. They all looked a little tired, though Jane in her 'Fun, Fearless, Female' T-shirt was certainly living up to the label. She had a cycling tan and the raised veins in her arms and legs were not a consequence of her treatment but through training.

Once the interview was finished, we dodged between the wetsuit-clad swimmers making their way down the stairs. I was extremely proud of all three girls, especially Rebecca who knew she'd probably finish last; but that had more to do with her having a crap bike than being a poor athlete. The previous week, she'd competed in a mixed age group bike race in Harrogate using an infant's bike with three gears, a small frame and knobbly tyres. She'd finished third out of five that day but today was much different. Seeing her legs spinning round the pedals while covering only half the ground she should have, was very amusing though we were careful not to laugh as she passed our vantage point. But it was hard for Steven and me to contain a snigger as she disappeared. We resolved to get her a new bike.

It was a relief to have all three safe and to be travelling home on the Sunday night. Suzanne had led the women in her age group for half the swim before her lack of training found her out. Rebecca thoroughly enjoyed the experience. Jane suffered in the extreme heat; her time was twenty minutes slower than the year before.

There were three weeks to the half ironman and I was becoming seriously concerned about her doing it. I'd watched her on as much of the course as I could and I thought she looked knackered during the run. She looked so uncomfortable that

135

I assumed it was inevitable she would drop out, but she grimaced and kept going. The half iron-man, which consisted of a 2 kilometre swim, 90 kilometre bike ride and half marathon, was twice the Olympic distance she'd just completed. Even just doubling the time would take her outside her target of seven and half hours.

The Sherborne Half Ironman had been this year's Holy Grail, though in truth it was only a staging post for the full ironman in Hawaii. Watching a video Mark Hayward had given Jane of the Hawaii Ironman featuring competitors with uncontrollable bowel movements losing con-sciousness and the brutality of the event had only seemed to inspire Jane. For me it only served to reinforce my belief that it was a mad event attracting only the sadistic. For a full ironman, seventeen hours was allowed, so Jane decided if she could complete Sherborne in seven and half hours then next year's Hawaii was achievable.

When you share a dream, it's surprising how many others buy into it and try to help. Mark, the PR man who'd given us the video, introduced Jane to his business partner Ryan, who gave her some tips about cycling the course. Mark also contacted some kit suppliers to try to upgrade Jane's equip-ment, which was very much at the cheap end of the scale. Of all the equipment she was going to need, the key item was the bike and through a contact they agreed to supply Jane with a carbon framed bike which would be substantially lighter than the aluminium one she was using at home. While this may seem a minor change, it could account for fifteen seconds a kilometre, and as

Jane would be cycling ninety kilometres, the total over the course could be significant.

We'd been amazed by the generosity that led to Jane's new bike but further treats were in store. One day at work Darren answered a phone call for me.

'Tommo, phone for you,' he said.

'Who is it, Daz?' His arm was outstretched as if the receiver was the Olympic torch.

'Posh southern accent, it'll be one of your media luvvies.'

'Piss off.' I walked past his arm, ignoring the phone. 'Will you put them through?' I asked, pushing away several project reports to clear some desk space.

I picked up the phone. 'Mike Tomlinson, Technology Leeds.'

'Mike, it's Karen at *GMTV* do you have a minute to talk?' My mind quickly flicked over why they would be making an unsolicited phone call and couldn't think of a reason.

'Yes, no problem.'

'You'll be aware that Concorde goes out of service soon. Well British Airways have donated a trip to New York on it, there's a week in a hotel included. We'd normally have it as a competition prize but we haven't got time to organise it. So we thought it should be given to someone who deserved a treat. Jane was suggested and we all thought what a great idea.' While she was talking I was quickly glancing around the office to check if anyone was struggling to contain a giggle. It seemed normal. 'What do you think? We wouldn't want anyone else to know, especially Jane. We'd come to your house live and surprise her.'

'Oh, I don't know what to say. I'm not sure it's something we could do without the children.'

'Sorry, I should have said; it's for all five of you.' I contemplated it for a moment again looking around; Karen and Mike had their earphones on, a couple of others were on the phone.

'I know this will sound churlish, it's a fantastic offer, thank you for thinking of Jane, but I need to have a think. Can I ring you back in fifteen minutes please?' I thought if I had their telephone number I could verify that it was *GMTV*.

'No it's our pleasure. Jane deserves it; she's done so much for others.' I hung up and stared at Darren.

'What?' he said.

'Are you bastards playing a practical joke?' I said quietly, trying not to attract the attention of the others to my potential paranoia.

'No.' He looked genuinely surprised by the question. 'Why?' I recounted the conversation. 'What are you going to do?' he asked.

'Phone Jane at work now.'

'I thought they said you weren't allowed to.'

'She was really pissed last year when I didn't tell her about the awards. Anyway who'd you be most scared of offending – Jane or *GMTV*? We just won't tell them she knows. It's not really practical not to tell her. She'll need to make sure she has permission from the hospital to travel. She'll have to cancel a treatment of Herceptin. Get the time off work. Sort out some travel insurance, which is impossible at the best of times.'

'Fair comment.'

'One question, do you think it'll affect the appeal?'

'What. How?'

'Taking a fantastic holiday, you know what people are like – even now a lot are sceptical.'

'Will it hell. Most'll say good luck; Jane deserves it. You don't though, I'll take your place.'

'You sure? If you think it will we just won't accept.'

'Not a penny, folks won't give a toss.'

JANE

We sat outside the café at Hampstead Heath and watched as the rain started to fall a little heavier. I was tired. We had been up early to go to the Sky studios in Isleworth and then all the way across London for an interview with ITN News. I had run a little way around the track on the heath, so that they could film me running, but was really frightened of doing too much stop-start running. All the hours' training could easily be wasted if I strained my back or leg muscles. So I had paced myself slowly round the track, running woodenly and without enthusiasm. It was a relief when the interview was over.

Now, sitting here watching the traffic buzz by, we were just finishing our lunch before travelling back across London to pick up the car and drive to Dorset. Suzanne had decided not to come with us, so there was just Rebecca, Steven, Mike and myself. As we drove across the country on the M4 we found ourselves staring at snakes of red tail-lights as cars heading towards the south-west all slowed down and stopped in the busy Friday afternoon traffic.

By the time we reached Taunton, the sun was starting to drop low in the sky, making it difficult to see the signposts. At last we came across the tall guesthouse in Sherborne, almost by accident. I sighed with relief. Mike was still fuming from the journey.

We lugged the boxes of equipment and the bags up two flights of stairs to the very top of the house and soon the immaculately prepared room was littered with bike spares, wet suit and other sundries for the Sunday coming.

'Do you fancy a walk out?' I asked Mike once Steven was settled in bed. Steven's blond hair stuck out in tufts and his eyes closed, the hollow of his cheek dipping in as he sucked at his fingers.

'Yeah, just for half an hour though.'

We walked down the cobbled main street past clothes shops and estate agents. Mike stood and looked at the boards in the windows.

Two short-haired men stepped out into the road to let us pass. As we drew alongside them, one turned to me. 'It is Jane, isn't it?' He thrust his hand towards me and I reached out to shake it.

'Mm, yeah.' I was dumbstruck and shook my head questioningly.

'It's great to meet you. What you are doing is fantastic.'

I smiled back at him. 'Thanks,' I said. 'Are you taking part this weekend?'

'Yes. I'm really looking forward to it.'

'Well,' I said, not knowing what else to say, 'have a great weekend, and good luck.'

'Good luck to you as well.'

We walked on and they continued on their way. 'Fame at last,' Mike said. I shook my head at him.

'That was weird,' I said, and we continued down the high street in our search for a pub.

At dawn on the Sunday, I left Mike, Rebecca and Steven sleeping in the room and crept downstairs where the lady of the house had risen to make me toast and coffee. I chewed on the toast but couldn't face any cereal or the bother of the crusts. 'Thank you,' I said as she bustled in and out of the kitchen. 'It was very good of you to do this. It's such an early start.'

I picked up my kitbag and slung it over my shoulder and headed for the door. The street lamps were still lit. The sky was just starting to lighten, but it was a dark, misty morning as I walked down the high street towards the castle. There were other athletes about stepping out nervously. Their bodies were tight; they clutched their bags with white-knuckled hands. We greeted each other with wide eyes and shook hands.

'Good luck. Have a safe one.'

As we made our separate ways to the starting area I walked with my head low, trying to keep myself calm. Once I had my goggles round my neck, my cap in my hand, I headed back to the queue by the Portaloo before joining the dark-skinned, seal-like crowd jostling each other to make their way into the water at the start.

I stepped on to the green carpet and down on

to the jetty and then lowered myself into the water. The stones under my feet were slimy with algae and duck poo. I shuddered and walked until it was deep enough to strike out with my slow breaststroke. I joined the bobbing bright hats as we trod water and tried to listen to the starter's instructions. My ears were covered by my swim cap, and I could barely hear the starter's voice as it ebbed and flowed like the tide. I shook my head but it made no difference. Then the hooter sounded and the water all around me turned white as 1200 people set off swimming at once, thrashing the water, making the mist rise white and thick from its surface.

MIKE

The last remnants of mist had cleared and the sun was forcing us to shed our extra morning layers of clothes. An eerie silence hung over the transition area where only two out of the 1200 bikes remained. Safety canoes were removing the swimmers' marker buoys and spectators were clearing the castle grounds, safe in the knowledge that even the quickest cyclists wouldn't be seen again for a couple of hours.

Lia, from the Press Association, had come down from York to cover Jane doing the event. Since the bike ride she'd been in regular contact with both of us and we were pleased to see her. We liked working with journalists we knew and could trust. Likewise Ian and Martyn were covering the event for Sky so it was a pleasant reunion. Martyn had

142

commandeered a bike but it was several inches too short for his six-foot frame. Watching him set off on the course to try to get some shots of Jane was rather amusing, his legs scrunched up like an adult on a child's bike. He said he would phone and let us know her progress.

'Can I take Steven to get a drink, Dad?' Rebecca asked. Normally I would have said no, but we were in a safe enclosed environment and they couldn't wander far. Even so I laid down a few rules.

'I'm fifteen not ten, Dad,' said Rebecca.

'You're my most precious things, so there can't be too many conditions.'

'Whatever.'

'I'll not be far away from here. I'll see you back at this spot in thirty minutes.'

'Yeah, yeah, yeah.'

'Relax, Mike,' Lia said. 'She's really sensible. You just don't see it because you're her dad. They seem so level-headed. The way they handle their mum being ill is fantastic.'

'They have their moments,' I said.

'Does Steven understand much?' Ian asked.

'His knowledge changes subtly over time as he becomes a little more inquisitive. He understands that there's just going to be the two of us at home. We joke that we'll get a season ticket for Chelsea. Now he understands that's never going to happen but it does reinforce the knowledge that mum won't be there.'

We set off on the path around the lake which had the double advantage of being both secluded and shaded. The occasional odd arrow or distance marker on a tree or fence was the only evidence that a sporting event was taking place. We walked on in silence until the path broke out into a clearing where the lake reappeared into view.

'I guess Jane being in the media makes it harder for the kids,' said Lia.

'Yes,' I said. 'Although they understand it's a necessary intrusion. I don't think the media's a big problem; we can shut ourselves off when Jane's not competing and they've mostly respected our privacy.'

'Most people in the media are really nice. It's just the odd one. But you get them everywhere,' Lia commented.

'The one major problem I can foresee is that after Jane's died I'll have a much bigger void to fill. It is going to be impossible for me to complete that maternal role but, because of the events, Jane's absence will leave a much bigger gap. With the events and fundraising they have such busy lives and suddenly they'll be empty. I'm not sure how that'll affect the children long term.'

I checked my watch and suggested we head back to meet Rebecca and Steve. Ian and Lia were quiet. Eventually Lia broke the silence, 'If there's anything I can ever do.'

'As it happens, I've been meaning to approach a subject when the time was right.'

'Go on.'

'It's really what to do when Jane dies.'

'What do you mean?' asked Lia.

'How to handle the media. I don't want people turning up at home and upsetting the kids.'

Ian looked across at Lia and said, 'It's probably

best to put a story out through PA wouldn't you say?'

Lia nodded. 'If we get some quotes it'll placate everyone. I'd be happy to do that. Just do that and then take the kids to stay with some relatives or friends. It only becomes a problem if people can't find details, the news is sketchy and they need to check facts.'

Ian said, 'Lia's right. You know plenty of people; we'll all help.'

It seemed such a tactless way to approach the subject but the reality was that one day it would happen and we would need to deal with it. My only concern was for the children. I didn't want them to be put under any more stress at what would undoubtedly be the most emotional time of their lives.

We completed the remaining part of the return journey in silence, the atmosphere hanging heavy. When we returned, Steven and Rebecca were playing without a care.

We were in exactly the same position four hours later while Jane was completing the second of her two laps of the run course. Jane's pledge – that if she completed the event in less than seven and half hours she'd train for a full ironman – looked like becoming a reality. As she was commencing her last lap, she needed only to complete the last ten kilometres in two hours, and that would be a formality.

We'd been joined mid-afternoon by my sister and her family as well as John Shanley from the charity SPARKS. Jane had completed the first half of the run in an hour so naturally we assumed that it would take longer for her to run the second half. But about forty-five minutes later, Martyn who had gone out to do a reconnaissance of the final couple of miles to ascertain Jane's position, appeared from the field pedalling furiously.

'Have you seen her?' Ian and I said in unison.

'It's fucking unbelievable,' panted Martyn. 'She was almost sprinting, she'd about a mile to go; she'll be here in a couple of minutes.'

The various news crews began to take up position and the guys from Sky were talking to their studio gallery, giving them an estimated arrival time so they could cover the finish live. I paced excitedly, I knew how much this meant to Jane, how much physical and emotional energy had been spent to get to this point.

'How long, Martyn? We're coming live,' said Ian.

'About two minutes.'

'No, she'll be at least five. I'll tell them to come to us in four,' Ian said.

'It'll be shorter than that, Ian, two minutes max at the speeds she's going.'

'Where did you see her?' Ian asked.

'She's here. She's here,' said Martyn pointing his arm. 'There, see, coming up the last hill, look at her fucking go. Fucking incredible!'

I shouted at the kids, 'Mum's here!' and like airmen scrambling for a plane, everyone jumped up and ran to get to the finishing line before Jane.

'Shit, shit, shit,' Ian mumbled desperately trying to get hold of the studio while also trying to get into a key position on the line to interview Jane as she finished. Two officials pulled a tape across the

146

finishing line especially for Jane, another stood in the wings with a bunch of flowers.

Jane beamed as she approached, she didn't look tired at all. In fact, her demeanour suggested she was competing a short Sunday afternoon training run, the supports on her knees the only evidence of someone carrying an injury. With twenty yards to go, she held her arms aloft, her face illuminated with unconfined joy. Eight months of hard work vindicated by a finishing time an hour ahead of plan. Ten minutes later and the media had disappeared like drinkers at closing time.

Jane looked at me. 'A full ironman it is then, next year Hawaii.'

'Are you sure you've not had enough? You couldn't even have imagined doing this in January and look how much it's taken out of you. Not just today. To double the distance, it's serious.'

'I know. But it's like when you've finished a half marathon, you just know it's not the real thing or even a quarter of it. Just a stepping stone. I know, with luck, I can do it – the full ironman. I know I can. I'll need some chemo, then "Rome to Home", then a full ironman.'

It would have sounded ominous, scary, terrifying, but as Jane stood, the top of her tri-suit unzipped, cheeks flushed, there was a steely determination in her voice that no one would have contradicted. 'I'm just going to collect my bike and wetsuit from transition.'

As she wandered away a group of ten people came over to congratulate her, their hands slapping her shoulder. I winced as I anticipated the pain that would cause her there – an area where the cancer was most prevalent. But she never flinched. After a quick hello to all of them, I watched her walk across the field – a solitary hobbling figure – and shook my head. She was so obstinate.

CHAPTER 5

September 2003

MIKE

With Suzanne leaving home for university the day after our return from New York, the trip would have extra resonance for all of us. Although Jane knew when and where we were going she didn't know when *GMTV* would surprise her. They had organised the time in advance with me to ensure it fitted in with their schedule and our normal daily routine and I'd sat in the living room with my friend Mick, who'd stayed over the night before, and Steven on the agreed morning to ensure the TV wasn't turned to channel three.

Five minutes before the time they were due to arrive and safe in the knowledge that Steven was engrossed in an episode of *Pokemon*, I went upstairs. Jane was fussing in the kitchen collecting sheets from the dryer, Suzanne was making sandwiches and Rebecca had already departed for school.

Despite a number of conversations with Karen

from *GMTV,* there was still a nagging doubt in my mind that we were being set up. That fear, however, was soon assuaged when I heard a commotion at the front door and Kate Garroway's husky voice barking into a microphone.

'Can you get the door, Suzanne, I'm getting dressed,' I shouted downstairs.

'No, I'm busy.'

'Mick?' No reply. 'Suzanne, where's your mum?' I asked.

'Pegging the laundry.'

'Mick?' I could hear shuffling in the living room. 'Suzanne, come on now,' I said authoritatively. I heard from the crew outside that they were running out of air time. My will wouldn't break first; at least they were getting the realism they'd asked for. Suzanne was first to give in. Within seconds the house had been invaded and we had the time of a commercial break to get organised. I crossed Suzanne on the stairs.

'You wazzock.'

'Is that any way to speak to your father?' I teased.

Downstairs, Mick was scurrying around departing the scene as quickly as he could, as though caught out by a returning husband. 'You arse,' he said. 'I fucking knew you were up to something.'

'Language, Timothy, there are microphones.' We squeezed passed each other in the hall and I gave a rueful smile.

'Arse,' he said again.

I'd primed Steven about Concorde travelling supersonic at twice the speed of sound; though it wasn't difficult as he has a passion for anything mechanical and fast. We'd tried to find a little book to buy which would be suitable for a small boy. Jane, too, was looking forward to going but there was some anxiety about whether we could organise travel insurance.

At the departure lounge at Heathrow there were dozens of passengers all waiting excitedly to board the majestic plane. Concorde appeared at the window, its nose bowed as if in reverence, and Steven gawped in wonder. His view was only temporary, though, as grown-ups pushed past him. People had paid huge sums for the privilege and weren't prepared to let a freeloading six-year-old hinder their desire to press their noses to the glass. I pushed my ankle-biter forward, instructing him to cause mayhem until he got to the front.

Concorde itself was a paradox; a supersonic aeroplane whose LED display was like something out of a 1960s sci-fi TV programme. It was as if its decline had been planned years in advance, knowing that a refurbishment would never happen. Quite how such a unique aeroplane could be allowed to cease flying was a mystery to everyone there.

By the time we arrived in New York at 7.30 p.m., roughly the same time we'd set off, we'd been up for eighteen hours and Steven was beginning to flag. When we stood on the roof of the Ritz Canton at Battery Park a few hours later, we'd all only managed six hours sleep in the last forty-eight.

A clock across the Hudson River advised us it was 1.30 a.m.; the statue of Liberty was a beacon on the near horizon. Jane clutched her back, stretching slowly.

'How are you feeling?' I asked.

'Fine,' she snapped. A semi-comatose Steven was down on the wall his head being cradled on Suzanne's lap. Two beautifully manicured lawns, whose grass was the vibrant green you'd see on a springtime Lakeland hill, looked like plastic. We were needed for a teaser at the head of *GMTV*'s programme before a couple of interviews. Steven was as upbeat as any six-year-old deprived of sleep.

'Show a little enthusiasm; we've brought you all the way to New York.' Kate Garroway tried to inspire the kids to display some artificial joy for a dress rehearsal interview. It invoked no response except a growl that Rebecca normally reserves only for me. As we went through the rehearsal Steven let his prop, a model of Concorde, slip through his fingers. Kate scowled at him and Rebecca at her. As the kids had done these live interviews countless times before they were treating the rehearsal and instructions with some contempt.

'Ten minutes to live,' the producer shouted. As if on cue, the sprinklers burst forth, showering not only the lawn but the equipment. Sensing a reprieve, we dispersed, while a mild panic distracted the crew. Hotel officials were scurrying around trying to work out what to do. No sooner was it under control than they lost connection with the satellite. Jane looked ill, for the first time in months her deterioration was visible.

We awoke next morning in a luxurious suite

151

overlooking Central Park. Outside, horse-drawn carriages vied with yellow cabs for space. New York smelled like walking into your grandma's kitchen, numerous sweet smells competing for your attention. The streets were busy, fast and unfriendly. Was there a place in the universe more alien to someone from a small market town in the Dales? I doubted it.

Knowing that it would be the last week we spent together – never mind the last family holiday – the trip weighed heavy on us; we knew it was time for Suzanne to leave but there was still sadness.

The TV crew was around for another couple of days and was excellent company without being intrusive, but it was good for the cameras to be put away.

JANE

After the grandeur and stunning views from the hotel opposite Central Park we thought we might be disappointed by the move across town to Battery Park, but we were welcomed to a very modern hotel with views across the Hudson to the Statue of Liberty. Around the corner was a small delicatessen with a dazzling array of fresh bread and prepared fruits.

With the Great North Run to complete on our return I was anxious not to lose my running fitness. I pulled on my running kit and took the lift down to the large lobby of the hotel. Pushing the heavy glass doors out on to the terrace I walked across the road to the Battery Park Esplanade. The grey block-paved surface was even and I ran with the black curling railings on my left. The dark surface of the Hudson River glinted now and then as the sun briefly emerged from behind clouds.

The pain in my back had started to increase, but as my feet fell the cramping and spasms lessened. I carried on past some tall columns and, intrigued, I made my way up the steps into yet another garden area. The pillars looked like some forgotten Greek temple. I ran until I came to the marina by the Winter Gardens – its vast glass atrium beckoning me to investigate.

I turned and passed the ranks of white yachts rocking gently at their moorings and made my way back towards the hotel, returning from my brief run feeling fresher in spirit if not in body. A man wearing a tall grey top hat pushed the door open for me.

'Good run, madam?'

'Yes, thanks. It was a great run.'

Across the lobby, I waited for the steel doors of the lift to slide open. Catching sight of my bed-raggled hair, the dark patch of sweat gathering at my neck, I stood self-consciously as others crowded into the lift, glancing curiously at me as they waited for it to make its smooth ascent.

Opening the door of our hotel room I could see Mike had made no effort to move from the bed. 'Do you know what we should do while we're here?'

Mike turned towards me, 'What?'

'We should go to a bar and have a Manhattan cocktail in Manhattan.'

'That would be perfect,' Mike said. 'Maybe

later tonight when Steven's gone to sleep.'

'I can't wait. Fantastic.'

The next morning, our suitcases were packed for our departure and the taxi stood waiting. The journey seemed much longer than it had to our sleep-deprived minds on the way out. It had been such an experience, so unexpected, now we were going back home.

'Where are you going to put everything?' I asked Suzanne, looking at the boxes and boxes piled in her bedroom. 'You won't get all of that lot in the car.'

I'd been looking forward to travelling over to Hull with her but it looked like I would have to make that trip another time. Her stereo and computer would take up the space that I might have sat in.

I looked down as Mike and Suzanne carried her belongings out to the car. 'Right, that's all we can manage,' Mike said.

Suzanne's face fell. 'But...' she started to say but changed her mind as she turned away from the car, her eyes narrowing. Controlling her temper, she stepped noisily back through the door, shutting it forcefully.

'Right, bye then,' she said as she gathered her coat around her.

'We'll see you soon.' I hugged her and she laid her head on my shoulder. Then she straightened herself up.

Smiling at me, 'I'll see you next weekend anyway,' she said.

'Oh yeah, I forgot.' I smiled back at her. 'Can't

154

even get rid of you properly.' She shook her head and stuck her tongue out at me.

'Come on, Suzanne.' Mike held the door wide for her. I stood and watched as he reversed out of the drive and drove slowly down to the main road. As he turned right, I waved and Suzanne waved back before the car disappeared from view.

I stepped back into the house and climbed the stairs. I stood in the doorway of her room. Emptied of its quilt, her bed looked naked. The whole room was bare. She had taken her pictures from the walls, her throws and cushions had all travelled with her. The warmth of her personality was gone. The curtains were open, but even the lazy evening sunlight couldn't lighten the room. It seemed dulled without her possessions, without her. She would be back but the house would be quieter without her. I knew I shouldn't be sad. I was lucky to have shared this goodbye with her, to see her move forward in her life. Our home still felt emptier.

MIKE

'How's Mum been?' Suzanne asked, as she wandered into the kitchen. I poured myself a drink, faking an interest in the label on the side of the carton, hoping it would buy me some time before I could give her an answer. I knew that if I told her the truth then she might feel guilty about moving away from home to university in Hull. But lying to her was not an option either.

'Oh, you know,' I said, bending over to put the

milk back in the fridge.

'No.'

'Coffee? How's uni?'

'Great, I'm really enjoying it.' Suzanne moved to the sink, clearing pots from the table as she passed it. 'You can't avoid the question. How's Mum?'

'Very fit, but if I'm honest she seems to be deteriorating. Earlier in the summer she was getting the odd bad day but now it's the majority of the time.' Suzanne's face momentarily flickered concern. 'Look, don't worry.'

'Will you phone me if you need me to come home?' she said, pushing her sleeves up and opening the dishwasher.

'You are joking,' I said.

'What?'

'We've been waiting years to get rid of you; we don't want you back after two weeks.' She flicked some moisture from the dishwasher at me. 'I'll run you back to Hull tomorrow night after I've finished work.'

Jane appeared, her cheeks flushed from a warm bath, but her movement was stiff and robotic like a Thunderbird puppet.

'Are you okay, Mum? Do you want a drink?'

'Chamomile tea, please.'

Suzanne took another mug out and flicked the kettle back on. 'Are you in much pain after the run?' she asked. 'Do you want to sit down and I'll bring it through?'

'I don't need to sit down,' said Jane. 'I'm not your dad.' She moved slowly across the kitchen floor and collected some clothes from the washer before brushing past Suzanne to gain access to

156

the dryer. 'Suzanne! I'm trying to get in here.'

'What?' Suzanne stomped away. 'I was only trying to help.' Jane loaded the tumble dryer. She could be quite precious sometimes about being in charge of the domestic chores and when her disease prevented her from doing them, it made life frustrating for all of us – for different reasons.

'Are you going to get a bath, Mike?' Jane asked.

'Yes.' I carried on reading the paper.

'You did well finishing in two hours fifteen,' she said alluding to my time on the Great North Run that afternoon. Her smugness at finishing half an hour ahead of me was evident from the smile that stretched across her face.

'Fuck off.'

'Oow. That's six minutes quicker than your personal best. Looooser.'

'Fuck off.'

We sat like book ends across the pine table. 'Don't do that, Mike,' Jane said as I sat using a pan lid to flick food crumbs that had got caught in a deep gorge that ran all the way across it. 'Did you miss your dad?' Last year's Great North Run had been his last day out before he was hospitalised.

'Yes, though I suspect I'd have been getting some stick now for losing so heavily to you. I miss not talking to him though, and I never get that sense that I will see him.' Jane looked at me quizzically. 'You know when you see someone who looks like somebody you know and then you realise it can't be because they are dead? That never happens. Maybe it's because it was so close a relationship, or maybe because I saw him die. Odd.' I sat meditating on his image, one of him

157

at Jane's big birthday party eighteen months ago.

'You haven't forgotten that I'm at hospital Tuesday have you?' Jane asked.

'How could I?' As the words left my mouth I knew they sounded harsh. It wasn't directed at Jane, it was just that I knew it would mean yet another three hours just waiting to see her consultant.

'There was nothing I could do about it,' Jane responded defensively. 'It's because I've asked to see them outside the normal review cycle. Is there anything you want to ask Dr Perrin?'

'No, how about you?' Experience told me that if there were ever to be a point that Jane would spring a surprise on me about her health, it would be now. How many times, almost as a passing phrase, had she advised me of a new area of disease, or that she'd been extremely ill or was particularly anxious? I looked across at her, studying any reaction that might betray a lack of openness.

'Nothing much really.' As usual it was the words that were not said that held the key.

'There's a "but" missing. What is it?' I asked.

'I've been getting increasingly dizzy, a clumsiness that makes even the simplest jobs difficult. Like constantly suffering from the effects of drinking four or five pints.' I looked disapprovingly at her. 'I didn't want you to be concerned. There was nothing you could do about it, apart from moan and tell me not to do the run.'

I let go an involuntary deep sigh. 'Is it time for chemo?'

'We'd already thought that this would be the time to ask for it but this just means that we don't have to make the decision. I don't want to wait and I think I'm mentally prepared to have a vigorous regime, something to hit it hard.'

'Okay.'

'It'll mean it finishes in plenty of time to do "Rome to Home". Hopefully it'll also buy sufficient time to get to Hawaii.'

When we arrived at the hospital there were about thirty patients waiting to see the consultant. From past experience, I knew we would be here a few hours. Dr Perrin is thorough and conscientious so while this means an inevitable wait it's well worth it. Because of his experience, there are often a number of people – including Jane – who ask for him specifically.

The waiting area is like an expanded doctor's surgery with two coffee tables surrounded by twelve wooden, low-seated chairs which have uniform blue upholstery matching chairs in adjoining rooms. In the corner is a 1980s-style, large Phillips TV whose only purpose seems to be to allow a fan to be placed on it.

The water cooler that once sat in the corner had gone. It had been removed when it became apparent that the bacteria in the water containers could actually be dangerous to patients on chemo. Tap water is safer for those with low immunities.

I picked up a copy of a glossy magazine and flicked through endless photos of celebrities whose only purpose in life was to ensure the pages were full. As I skimmed through the pages, my irascibility increased and I swapped it for a badly printed women's magazine. A collection of non-celebrities were complaining about how life had dealt them a rum hand. I threw it back; drivel, a table full of absolute nonsense. I slid down the chair slightly and rested my head against a dado rail.

'Mike, Mike.' I opened my eyes and looked at Jane. 'You'd drifted off.' I rubbed my eyes and checked the clock. It was 3.20 p.m. I looked around the room; there was no discernible difference in either the numbers or occupants of the chairs. Sue Hector, the IV room sister, was stood talking to Jane.

'That was cruel, Jane,' she said.

'No more than he deserves. He either spends his time complaining of being tired or asleep.'

Sue looked at me. 'You can go in the IV room if you like, Mike. Most of the chairs are empty; we're just finishing the last few patients.'

It was an afternoon upgrade akin to going from cattle class to first class on a plane and I jumped at the opportunity. Jane had a disgusted look which said: 'Don't indulge him', but by then I was moving out of earshot quicker than I had done on the Great North Run.

'Mike, Mike,' a soft voice spoke. Slowly I recovered my bearings and realised it was Sue Hector.

'Mike, get up. The staff want to go home.' I looked at the window and it was already pitch black.

Re-emerging into the waiting room I noticed that we were the only people left. Within minutes though we were sat having a consultation with Dr Perrin. After an overview of Jane's current symptoms, Dr Perrin leafed through Jane's notes: scans, treatments, Jane's previous symptoms, pausing occasionally to study a page in detail. He examined Jane, pushing against her stomach; presumably to discover any pain in her vital organs, but what did I know. After he sat back down he asked Jane what was her opinion of her current situation.

Jane had always been in a much better position to advise the doctors on her current state of health than the scans, which always seemed to have a time lag of three to twelve months.

Dr Perrin said, 'Are there any indications of your disease advancing?'

'I'm having increased pain in my back and ribs. I'm also beginning to feel dizzy, unbalanced at times.'

Dr Perrin looked at her. 'We'd better have a quick look, Jane.' She climbed on to the bed while he closed the curtain. I pulled my reading book from my fleece pocket to try to release my tension. Eventually, after the physical examination they returned to their seats and Dr Perrin explained the treatment options to Jane.

Choosing a treatment for terminal cancer is like looking into a virtual medicine cabinet. Only a certain number of treatments are stacked on the shelves and once you take one out, it's never restocked. Once a chemotherapy has been used, its effectiveness on a second occasion is reduced.

Treatments vary – their toxicity, effectiveness, side effects – choosing one is a delicate balance between quality of life and benefit to your immediate health. If your health is good generally,

161

you wouldn't choose a highly toxic one, for instance.

But unusually, because Jane had been on a course of it before, Taxotere was offered again. It was three years since she'd first had it – then in conjunction with Epirubicin – and their joint effects had resulted in Jane's health improving dramatically. She'd stood on the precipice of death so it wasn't a decision to be treated lightly, but at its mention it seemed the drug of choice – for all of us.

Dr Perrin has an ability to make you believe you are making a choice, but always during a quiet reflection later it's apparent that by his influence you've been steered like sheep into a pen. Sometimes it's good to be led.

JANE

I swallowed the four small white tablets, washing them down with milk and grimacing as they stuck in my throat. Working my mouth, trying to force them further down towards my stomach, they eventually slipped down. I had only taken two doses of steroid, but already my eyelids felt swollen, my cheeks puffed out.

I filled the kettle and clicked it on to boil, dreading how I would feel later. These small delays would put the treatment off just a little longer.

Mike placed his empty cup down. 'Come on then, we'd better get off.'

Reluctantly, I picked up my bag containing the sandwiches I'd made earlier as well as a bottle of water and my book and headed to the car.

I sat for a long time in the waiting area at the oncology unit. The backrest of the blue chair was digging into the small of my back and I couldn't get comfortable. I shuffled about until finally it was my turn. Catherine the nurse stood at the door.

'There's a chair free now at the end on the right,' she said and I made my way into the treatment room.

Four hours later and my eyelids were heavy, my mouth dry. Fighting nausea, I clutched my coat around me and headed for the toilet. The needle had been taken out and I could move about once more, unencumbered by a drip stand and infusion set. I swayed unsteadily back to the chair and started to gather up my belongings. 'Right, I'm done,' I said to Mike, my voice lowered with tiredness.

As soon as we arrived home I grabbed a glass and filled it with water. Longing for a drink, I could force only a few sips down through my dry cracked lips.

'I'm off to bed,' I muttered and, clutching the glass, made my way up the stairs. I lay still listening to the clanks and bangs from the kitchen below as Mike started to make the evening meal. I could hear the click, click, click, click of the faulty automatic ignition on the cooker oven. I closed my eyes and the darkness deepened. Sweat gathered on my face and I reached for a small hand towel to wipe it away. Much later I woke, my body felt heavy. I could make out the street lights through the curtain reflecting from the picture at the end of the bed.

Over the next few days, I managed to crawl out of bed to eat and drink and slowly I started to feel less nauseous. By Sunday, I even managed a short walk around the local park, but soon became exhausted. In bed that night I turned on my right side, the cramp and muscle spasms under my ribs making me so uncomfortable. The pain in my back and thighs made me feel stiff and I sat upright to turn myself again.

I lay on my back in the darkness. My eyes closed, the sparkle and fizz of the remembered light on my eyelids. Light greens and airy purples, there was one bright spot just above the centre of my vision. Behind my closed eyelids I followed the small sparks of light chasing it upwards with my eyes, but no matter how I tried I could not lift it higher than the top of my unsighted field.

Tiring of that, I opened my eyes but could not make out the forms in the bedroom. The red dot distant at the end of the bed showed where the radio was. The fireworks from my eyes moved ceiling-ward as I rested my head back against the pillow. I waited for my eyes to adjust to the darkness and the room to gather itself properly once more around me.

The remnants of light moved higher, but now they seemed to be obscured by the darkness rather than fading. Black shapes seemed to have angular wings. As I lay there I could feel the blackness pushing heavily down on me, feel the formless night swooping towards me. My hands were placed either side of my head on the pillow. As I watched the blackness moving in closer

closer towards me I could feel it reaching out to touch me. My breath gasped out and then in, then I held it again, trying to hear any sounds out beyond my covers. I crept my hands downwards till they were protected by the covers, pulling the quilt up to the bottom of my nose. The darkness moved closer, hung heavier, as I eased myself up and turned to my left side to try to stop the blackness surrounding me.

On my side, I could make out the light behind the curtains of the two bedroom windows. But instead of comforting me, tonight the windows, black edged with yellow, seemed like the eyes of some great beast gazing dozily through the walls of my house.

I shut my eyes tight and blew air between my lips. A slow, steady stream. My heart was thumping and I gasped a breath in trying to slow it down. I blew out once more and drew a more controlled breath in and out till I felt calmer.

I watched the room from beneath my covers, trying to gain enough courage to leave my bed. Then with one more breath I dashed back the covers and swung myself out of bed. I made it to the door. It creaked as I opened it cautiously. Once I was on the other side of it I closed it quietly and stood on the landing.

The bathroom door was open and light from outside shone through the bathroom, dimly lighting the hall. I crept downstairs and turned towards the kitchen. The door protested as I opened it, trying my hardest to be quiet. I reached my hand in and pushed down the switch. At once, this darkened land of shadows was harshly lit. The naked light bulbs of the kitchen cast their harsh light, bouncing off the kettle and the glass kitchen door units. My lids closed slightly while my eyes adjusted to the light.

The kettle finished hissing and bubbling and I slowly filled the mug, watching the tea bag turn from opaque white to transparent so I could see the yellow-green chamomile leaves and flowers. I left the kitchen light on but closed the door behind me and opened the one to the living room, turning on the small lamp.

I pulled the rug from the back of the settee. I curled my legs underneath it and wrapped my cooling body with the familiar blue blanket, moons and stars picked out in yellow. My head rested back against the settee as I took tiny sips of my tea, blowing across the top to try to cool the herbal brew quicker.

I swallowed the last of the calming tea and held the still warm mug against the side of my neck, enjoying the heat radiating from it. At last it was too cool to savour any longer and I reached out and placed it on the large square pine table. The flat expanse was covered with the debris of the evening. Power Ranger toys in bright blues, yellows and reds. Mike's side plate from his late night snacks. Sunday papers and supplements lying in scrunched heaps.

My hand rested against the small dark box. Almost black, the shiny lacquered surface dragged against my fingers, the smoothness and polish nearly hiding the purple colour. Its small slightly domed top on the lozenge-shaped body made it look like one of the capsules I swallow down each day in an effort to control my cancer. I brought the box towards me and cradled it between both hands, feeling the smoothness, the warmth of the wood beneath its dark cold exterior. I slowly pushed open the lid and the orange-yellow untreated wood was like a wound slicing open the finish.

The interior held some battered photographs. They were all in colour, faded – the yellows too bright, the greens too dull. I lifted the small collection out and looked at them one by one.

A young lady with long blonde hair, dark at the roots, pale faced, her eyes surrounded by dusky purple shadows. Suzanne's face is a little fuller – a little older – and there I am, sitting next to her, perched on a white sheet of a hospital bed. My hair is peppered with grey around the temples, my face more creased. My eyes are fully open and my lips are turned up in a large smile. In my arms, a small white-wrapped bundle. A tiny glimpse of dark downy hair is visible. Suzanne's hand reaches out to touch and own her baby.

In the next snap, Mike stands dressed in a sombre suit. White crisp shirt and a grey tie. At his shoulder is Rebecca, her hair curled and swirled around her head, held back by a small silver tiara, little crystals dangling down to her forehead. The white dress is tight across her breast and her arms make a triangle across her front, her hands obscured by a bouquet of white roses, with some delicate dusky pink blooms contrasting against the dark small-leaved ivy. Her smile sits tight on her lips, her eyes wrinkled at the edges where the anxiety is creasing her face. Mike looks relaxed next to her, as if he has been caught in conversation with the photographer.

The next photo is slightly larger. I can make out the edges where it has been cut from a group of four identical pictures. Steven's round face is surrounded by a shock of light brown hair. The fringe sits wildly across his forehead, the tufts hidden under the dark square of the mortar board, the tassel dangling, the fringed end tangled. The dark gown hangs awkwardly to one side. His smallish white hand holds it in place and his other hand holds the white scroll. He looks up at the camera from under the brow of the board. His eyes squint slightly, but a smile is flashing across his face. He looks like he's doing a duty and is anxious to be off with his mates.

The last picture is small and round-edged with an ancient yellow blob of glue on the back. It's the picture from an estate agent's house brochure. The colours are muted. The white cottage looks like it's smiling. Two windows beneath a dark slated roof sit above two larger ones resting either side of a big slated porch supported by wooden pillars. The heavy dark-wooded door is shut. The letterbox is a grin across the door. At the side a roof slopes down on a blank white wall into a dry-stone-walled garden. The greys and browns of the haphazardly laid stones reach just above the sills of the windows.

If you could open the door you would find a grey-blue slate floor. An ancient mat that many shoes and boots have had the underneath scoured on. A cardboard box advertising some sugary child's drink is filled with green and red Wellington boots. Above the boots there is a heavily laden coat rack, small, medium and large blue and green waterproofs draped

168

down the wall.

From the hall you can see through the door into the kitchen. Warm-coloured terracotta tiles against an old scratched cooker. A pine table is just visible, with newspapers strewn across it. The house would echo with laughter and the buzzing of voices. The voices could be chattering, arguing, angry, crying. Mostly its just family voices but friends as well. Many people have passed between this door, walked the hills around and enjoyed a beer at the table, warmed themselves in the small snug at the furthest end of the house. It's a house full of memories. Memories I'll never have, arguments and jokes not shared, friendships ended and no longer enjoyed.

I gathered up the collection of photos and put them back into the purple-black box, closing the lid carefully on the future I won't experience. Leaning back, cradling the box against me, enclosing it with my arms and my body, I rested my head against the settee, my neck long and white, the better to swallow the bitter pill. I worked my mouth, my tongue, the better to force the memories down, pushing the blackness of them deep into the centre of myself.

The darkness of that night followed me through the next few days. It was hard to lift my mood. My anxieties about the future hung heavily over me. The chemotherapy left me feeling tired and the cramps and muscular aches caused by the drugs exacerbated my pain.

I was tired when we arrived in London. My face looked yellowish through illness and I had struggled to sleep through the night, waking weary and irritable in the morning. I had showered in the small bathroom of our hotel room, smeared moisturiser on my face and brushed my hair gently so as not to remove too much hair – it was already starting to fall out. I outlined my eyes and put some colour on my cheeks, brightened my eyes with shadow and filled in my lips with lipstick. Helen Sykes in Armley had given me a beautiful white suit. I eased the skirt over my narrow hips and zipped it closed, smoothing it down. Sliding my feet into elegant high shoes, I tried on the tall navy and white hat. Try as I might, I couldn't get it to sit elegantly on my head, it kept sliding to one side, looking rakish not sexy.

Finally, I was satisfied. With Mike dressed in his suit, we met Suzanne and Becca in the lobby of the hotel and ordered a taxi to our friend's workplace. Cassie had agreed to look after Steven while we went to Buckingham Palace. I wished Steven could be with us, but I was only allowed to bring three guests, no more under any circumstances.

Sitting carefully in the taxi we watched London slide by outside and finally we arrived at the Palace. A snaking queue of smartly dressed people was waiting to pass through the security. Cars pulled up and waited to be inspected before being allowed to carry on through into the gravelled drive of the Palace.

I handed the passes over to the police officer.

'Have you got a letter with you as well?' he asked.

My eyebrows raised. 'No. That's all I've brought.'

'Oh. What name was it?'

'Jane Tomlinson and this is my family here.'

The police officer stepped back and conferred with his senior officer. They both glanced through sheets of paper on clipboards.

'That's fine. If you follow that queue there.' He pointed to a steady stream of people moving towards the Palace. 'Someone will let you know where you need to go.'

We did as instructed and I turned to kiss Mike goodbye as we separated at the entrance and I climbed wide steps to the long elegant hall. Original oil paintings of pictures I'd only seen as reproductions hung along it and everybody stayed by the edges, unsure what to do or who to speak to.

I took a glass of orange juice from the tray offered and sat on a cushioned seat on the edge of the room. Tired and my legs shaking, I watched as people started to clump together. A woman behind me asked what I was there for.

'And what are you being honoured for?' I asked her. She, too, was involved in charity work.

A tall man glided into the room, clearing his throat. 'Can I have your attention?' he called clearly across the long room. We all fell quiet and listened as he explained how we must curtsey and then step back from the Queen as well as what to expect from the honours ceremony.

'Her Majesty has a very firm handshake and you will know when it is time to step back,' he said.

We craned our necks to watch a video which demonstrated the correct etiquette and soon it was time to line up. Our names were called and we were processed slowly through the hall, waiting to be directed to the next room. It felt like a school prize-giving night or a graduation ceremony.

I followed everyone else and walked along the outside of the next room till a hand rested on my shoulder, indicating for me to stop and wait for my turn. Then I was eased forward.

'Enjoy the moment,' the gentleman said into my ear and I stepped into the room with two thrones and walked up to the dais where the Queen was raised above me.

'So you run do you?' she asked as she pinned the badge to my suit. I felt I towered over her, not something I experience often as I am petite. My tongue stuck to the top of my mouth and I was unable to respond. I felt my hand being shaken and then pushing me back and I turned and walked to the back of the hall where a man pointed to a space in the row of seats. I slid quietly into a chair and watched as others came forward to be honoured.

Afterwards, out in the courtyard, I shivered in the chill autumn wind as we waited for the photographs. Familiar faces from various news programmes were there to speak to me so it was a long time before we are able to leave. Sting and Roger Moore, who I had spotted earlier, were no doubt already celebrating with family and friends at upmarket restaurants in London. Mike and I walked out of the Palace back towards Westminster to pick up Steven and enjoy a sandwich at the head office of the SPARKS charity I support.

'Jane, do you mind waiting?' Dave the reporter

for Yorkshire Television asked. 'We'd like to speak to you live in about fifteen minutes.'

Before I could say anything, Mike replied for me. 'Of course we don't mind, we've nowhere else to go.' I stared at him as we stood outside the palace gates. All the other guests had left and would be celebrating their honour, somewhere. We were still here, not for ourselves but for the media who wanted to show an ordinary person receiving an honour. My feet ached from the unfamiliar height of the dress shoes.

'Don't bother asking me what I might want to do!' I snapped at Mike. His face froze, the smile fixed on his face.

'Don't carry on. It's hardly inconvenient waiting fifteen minutes, and it will help the charities. You know it will,' he said.

'Perhaps I'd like a day that was about me and not the charities,' I said turning away from him, towards Dave, who directed me to a spot that would show Buckingham Palace in the background. I forced a smile on my face.

Back at the hotel I changed out of my beautiful white suit and placed the hat back into the box. I put on my loose trousers and huddled myself into a baggy jumper ready to sit in the car for three hours for the return journey home. My head hurt and I rubbed my hand against the back of my scalp. As I did so, a large clump of hair came away. I balled it up between my hands and looked for a bin.

'My hair's definitely falling out now,' I said to Mike as we sat in the car watching the traffic moving slowly in front of us.

'You looked beautiful today,' he said. I looked out of the window and swallowed back a sob. 'Are you going to shave your head?'

I nodded and wiped the tears from my eyes. I couldn't face losing my hair but there was nothing I could do about it now.

MIKE

I climbed out of the bath, which once again I'd run too hot causing my head to spin as I took some tentative steps. Entering the bedroom Jane was applying some foundation, mirror in front of her, dress laid out perfectly across the bed. Her cheeks were bloated from the steroids, her head bald from chemo, eyebrows gone. I could see her eyes strain to focus, her right hand grappled for a cotton bud; her complete concentration was required for the simplest of tasks.

'Are you okay?' I asked. There was no reply so I continued with the obstacle course that was our bedroom, repositioning the rocking chair, climbing over a suitcase to access the wardrobe and liberate my monkey suit.

'Will this dress be okay, Mike?' she turned and waited for my answer. I was acutely aware that this was the first public function Jane had attended while bald. Three years ago when she'd lost her hair, Jane had never even done a run so our lives were completely private.

'Yes, you'll look lovely as always.'

'Mike, don't patronise me and trot out pat answers.'

174

'Okay, what are the alternatives?' I asked.

'There's this or the one I wore last year.'

'Well at least that makes your decision easy.' Jane's eyes closed involuntarily as she raised her hands to her mouth and yawned. Her movements were sluggish, clumsy like a punch-drunk boxer. 'Did you manage to get a rest this afternoon?'

'I tried,' she said. 'But my back was too sore; I just couldn't get into the right position.'

'We don't have to go tonight,' I said. 'People will understand. You're on chemo. Your last treatment was eight days ago. No one would expect you to suffer for going to it.'

In truth I'd been dreading tonight's Yorkshire Awards. A couple of months previously I'd been advised that the awards committee wanted to recognise my efforts with the appeal with a special award, similar to the one Jane had received the year before. My initial instinct was to say, thank you, but no thank you. I'd been nominated for a similar award earlier in the year and I'd found out because the BBC had telephoned me at work. I told them that, while I was immensely flattered, I didn't want to be recognised.

When Jane had heard what I'd done she was incensed. 'You hypocrite,' she said over dinner that night. 'I've been going to award ceremonies for a year.' She began to mimic my voice, 'You need to accept it; it's good for the charities, Jane, increases the profile. We'll raise more money, Jane. If you don't go the charities will lose out, Jane.'

I put my knife and fork down. 'What good is me getting an award,' I asked. 'That's not going to benefit anyone.'

Jane had sternness to her face. 'Let's put it this way. You'll ring the BBC tomorrow and accept the nomination.'

'But–'

'No buts.'

'Yeah, Mum, go for it,' Suzanne roared encouragement. 'Don't let him wheedle out of it, the scumbag.'

'Yes, Mum, not fair it is,' Steven chipped in.

'If you don't go, I won't attend any more award ceremonies, dinners or charity do's. You'll have to get permission to set up interviews. There might not even be any more events.'

While I didn't doubt Jane's seriousness, I detected that there was an element of her revelling in this. 'If I hear you've declined any award at any stage in the future it's the end of the appeal.'

So two months later I was told I'd been nominated to receive a special recognition award at the Yorkshire Awards. I'd not told Jane so she wouldn't feel obliged to go. Jane drew on all her reserves to ensure she attended. By design, we arrived as late as possible at the champagne reception to ensure Jane wasn't on her feet for too long. I stood like a wallflower as various people came up to her. She flashed each one with a smile, chatted nonchalantly and dismissed any concerns over her health.

Five hours later it was with some relief that I could unhook my trousers and allow my girth to expand to its natural size. I quickly changed into jeans and T-shirt as even though it was late, I didn't feel like bed.

Jane came in with a flannel to discard the war

paint. She had managed well at the awards ceremony until about 10 p.m. and then she started to flag. Although there was no discernible difference to anyone else, I saw the telltale signs straight away – her left eye half shut, losing posture, the odd wince of pain.

'How long had you known?' she asked.

'What?'

'Don't be obtuse, Mike. The award. How long had you known about the award?'

'Not long. Do you want a coffee?' I made a move to exit the bedroom.

'How long? Clearly Steve, Darren and Kevin knew.' There had been a couple of interviews from friends on the screen at the ceremony but they were a surprise to me as well.

'They didn't know I knew. We never discussed it.'

'How long?'

'One to two months.'

'We'll say two months then shall we?' she said. 'But you never thought about telling me in all that time.'

'It wasn't important.'

'Not important. You tell me whether Chelsea have won every match and all kinds of trivial rubbish.'

I shuffled around at the door, unsure what to say. 'I did think about telling you but didn't want to pressure you into going,' I said.

Jane stood up. 'Bollocks, absolute bollocks. If you ever do that to me again, ever, I'll walk out of the room. I made it absolutely clear that if you kept secrets like this, then I'd not go to any more.' I motioned to move away. 'Stop. Have I made myself clear?' she said in a very head-mistressy tone.

'Actually what I agreed was that if you were to get any more awards which were a surprise, I'd tell you. Clearly this wasn't the case here.'

'Do not,' she said, wafting the flannel in my general direction, 'take the piss and split hairs. You knew the intention of the words I said; don't twist the meaning like a lawyer.'

'Okay. Whatever.' I tried to give her a hug.

'Don't "whatever" me and don't bloody touch me.'

'Did you say whether you wanted a coffee?'

'Please.'

I moved closer and held her. The extra weight she was carrying was noticeable but more signifi-cantly she slumped down, allowing me to take a share. She was as exhausted as if she'd done a marathon, every ounce of energy had been given in today's seventeen hours of work, shopping, family and tonight.

'Congratulations anyway, you've deserved it,' she said.

There must have been plenty of cold, damp miserably wet days in Settle when I was a child but I don't remember them. I can only start to recollect them from mid teens, when they are all I can recollect. Jane jokes that even during a drought it rains the moment she arrives in Settle.

Jane was due to switch on the Christmas lights tonight on the marketplace in front of the Shambles, the centre of town, and the weather wasn't being considerate.

'Come on, Steven, put your coat on.' My mum was fussing over him, holding out his coat behind his back.

'Do we have to?' Steven slotted his arms in as if he was doing his grandma a favour.

Once in, he moved back to the seat which Becca had just pinched to continue watching the half-time football scores. Becca hit the red button on the remote, turning the television off. 'Aww, I was watching that,' said Steven. Rebecca smiled and tossed the remotes on to the floor further away from him. He moved to collect them so she stood up and body-checked him.

'Hey! Did you see that – he just kicked me?' she squealed. Mum and I turned round and Steve smiled at us angelically. There was a creaking from the stairs and, seconds later, the door to the hall opened slowly and Jane appeared, looking groggy from her afternoon rest. The debilitating effect of the chemo and the need for relief from the constant pain meant she always tried to rest her body mid-afternoon – without it she suffered in the evening.

'Are you okay? Do you want some help?' I asked.

'Shut up, Mike.' Jane was always grouchy after waking up, whatever the time of day it was. She didn't like to be talked to first thing; I suppose I should have known better. For the first couple of years of our life together I'd taken her barbed responses personally but now I was used to them.

Even so, on this occasion, my pride was dented. 'It's good to see you too,' I said.

'Shut up. For God's sake, stop droning on.'

'Come on, we need to get going,' I urged. But Jane was one-paced so we all sat waiting with our coats and watched her go through the routine: medicine, shoes and coat. I could sense she was frustrated at us waiting, so I spirited Steven to the kitchen and then to the back step.

Outside the bristling cold air had us all tugging our hats an extra few centimetres down our heads. My mum fussed, checking the house, making slow inexorable progress before finally closing the back door. 'Come on, Mum, it's freezing.' She wouldn't be rushed though. As we set off, I lagged back with my mum, walking shoulder to shoulder, while a little way ahead Jane was on the outside of Steven holding his hand. Rebecca had shot off and was a couple of hundred yards ahead just like her granddad would have been.

'Are you sure you won't come to ours for Christmas?' I asked my mum.

'I'm sure.'

'You shouldn't be on your own.'

'I'm on my own every day,' she said, though not with bitterness. 'I'll go to Age Concern's dinner at St John's.'

The thought of my mum going to get a charity Christmas dinner didn't sit comfortably with me, but this was just my own stigma. I knew she would enjoy having a meal with lots of people she knew well and not having to fuss cooking for one. But it did nothing to help me feel better about leaving her alone. I'd been observing how Mum had coped since my dad's death without approaching the subject directly. She'd said nothing, but there'd been an obvious tiredness every time we'd seen her. Jane had commented frequently on how she was looking tired but I felt unqualified to do anything.

For me, returning home to an empty house, especially during winter, is a scary glimpse into my own family's future. Occasionally, someone will ask me whether I've contemplated life without Jane. It's a question best ignored.

'Anyway the offer's there and I know Janet's asked you down to Torquay. I'd quite fancy the English Riviera as opposed to the cold here,' I said.

We made our way in silence to the Naked Man Café, where we were met by the organising team. While we sipped tea and munched mince pies, Jane went to perform her official function.

'Are you going to watch, Michael?' my mum asked.

'No.'

'Come on.'

'Just leave it, will you.' I'd never got used to hearing Jane being introduced to the public, the pain never lessened each time her host reminded everyone about the 'terminal cancer'. I could envisage Jane stoically listening and smiling, her mind numbed as she was told she was dying again.

I could see the crowds outside grow steadily. After the countdown, the town's illumination and fireworks over Castlebergh, I knew Jane's duties would be over. I donned my hat and headed out with Steven to get a good view of the pyrotechnics. I looked across the heads of people and thought how proud my dad would have been.

181

I wandered through the people, hoping no one would recognise me. I was happy that people wouldn't remember me from my school days or working at the garage; a past life best forgotten. I looked at Jane across the marketplace and I felt I'd already lost a part of her, she was in a place I couldn't imagine or reach, like watching a film I'd started to share her with strangers. I tugged Steven's arm and set off to join her, deeply saddened by my recent loss – and my future one.

CHAPTER 6

January 2004

JANE

The snow blew towards us, stinging our faces, then the wind dropped and the hard white flecks seemed to hang in the air before floating towards the ground. Just before they settled, the wind built up again and Melissa, Suzanne and I bobbed our heads down, tucking our chins into the top of our coats and pulling our scarves up over our mouths.

The pub was noisy and crowded when we arrived and had no seats left. We squeezed alongside the bar towards the rear and the games room. I stood behind two men leaning against the bar, their tall pint glasses in hand waiting to be served.

'You can squeeze in here, love,' said one and moved just slightly to the side allowing me to access to the bar. The British Oak was a loud merry place, especially on New Year's Eve. People were chatting loudly, friends were hailing each other across the pub. The deal was that we – the girls – went out first, leaving Mike; Melissa's husband, Steve; Mick and Tom, Suzanne's boyfriend, at home looking after the kids so they could come out afterwards. I ordered three drinks and carried them back to Suzanne and Melissa.

'So,' said Melissa, taking her glass. 'Are you and Luke sorted for the big bike ride then?'

'Hopefully,' I said, raising my voice a little to make myself heard. 'We're just starting to think about it seriously now.'

'Whereabouts are you cycling?'

Suzanne had been listening and joined in the conversation. 'They're starting off at Rome and heading up through Italy and France to Leeds. Yeah,' said Suzanne, noticing that Melissa's eyebrows were raised in disbelief, 'she IS mad.'

'I take it you are cycling with Luke again?' Melissa asked.

'Yeah, that's right. I don't envy him. Five weeks with me on the road.'

'What on earth do you want to do that for?' asked Melissa.

'Well we want to do something similar to John o'Groats to Land's End to raise money, but we want it to feel a little more isolated than we were on that trip.'

'So whereabouts are you going?'

'I've not sorted out the route properly yet but fancy going through Siena, Florence and the road into France and up to Paris. I've still got to

183

buy the maps and plan it all properly.'

'That will take some time,' she said.

I took a sip and nodded. 'It's hard work – looking at maps all day till you see the best route, but it's worth it and we can always change where we're going to en route.'

We carried on chatting, with Melissa telling me about the latest news on her extension. Steve and Melissa had been married nearly as long as Mike and me. I'd known Steve as long as I'd known Mike. We had a tradition of celebrating New Year's Eve together. My house was always the venue. Christopher and Daniel were close in ages to Steven, so it was a night for everyone to enjoy.

After what seemed like only half an hour but was more like two, Suzanne suddenly looked concerned. 'Is that the time?' she asked.

I glanced over my shoulder and looked at the clocks then checked my watch. 'Twenty past ten. We'd better get moving so the blokes can get out for a drink.'

We glugged the last of the beer from the bottles and Melissa lifted her golden half of cider and took another sip. We stood and squeezed ourselves into our warm outdoor clothes and pushed our way back out of the pub.

The wind had dropped and the snow was only coming down in small flakes now, but we hurried along the road. At the house, we pushed the door open and the sounds of the television and Steve and Mike's voices could be heard from the living room.

'Has Steve tucked in Chris and Danny?' Melissa asked with a glint in her eye.

Steve appeared from the living room and ambled down the hall. 'I'll just get my shoes on and we'll be off for some refreshments,' he said. Mike appeared at the doorway as well. He put on his fleece. As he pulled his hat from his pocket a cloud of tissue floated on to the floor. Mike, Mick, Steve and Tom wrapped themselves up and made their way out.

'Shut the door,' Suzanne called. Relative peace was restored.

'Aah, that's better,' Melissa said as she sat down.

The cooker timer beeped and I put on my oven glove and opened the oven door.

'Is there any sign of them yet?' I said. Suzanne opened the front door and peered down the road.

'Nope, not yet.' She turned to close the door.

Seconds later, however, they appeared breathless in the kitchen. Mick had one very pink ear and Mike's coat had a large patch of snow on the back. Tom appeared unscathed. Steve turned, threatening us with a ball of fresh white snow he was patting round in his hands.

'You can get that outside,' Melissa warned, watching from the settee in the living room.

'Yes, sir.' Steve drew himself to attention and tossed the snowball through the open front door.

'I thought you were going to miss midnight,' I said to Mike.

'You know I'd never do that, my love.' Mike grinned at his mates. 'I wouldn't dare.'

He shrugged his shoulder away from me as if fearful I would assault him. He didn't know just how close he came to being belted, but I drew a breath and turned back to removing the mini pizzas, samosas and sausage rolls from the oven, tossing them from the hot oven dish to plates on the table. I climbed up on to the kitchen top, balancing precariously, and stretched up to reach the champagne flutes in the far corner. Passing them to Suzanne, I made my way unsteadily down to the chair and back on to the floor.

Jools Holland was counting down to midnight as I returned to the living room with the bottles and glasses, so I eased the cork from one bottle and Suzanne popped the cork open from the other and we hastily poured the golden bubbles into glasses and handed them around. Everyone lifted their glasses as people danced and kissed strangers on the television. We all made our way around the room, hugging and exchanging New Year greetings and kisses with friends and family as well as our neighbours Cynthia and Terry.

'Happy New Year, everyone,' Mike shouted as Rebecca opened the patio doors and stepped out into the back garden. As the cheering on the television died down we listened to the thunder and watched the bright lights flowering in the sky heralding in the year 2004.

MIKE

Back in 2000, when it was thought that Jane had less than six months to live, Kevin, my boss, had kindly offered me some sabbatical leave until Jane died, although I didn't take him up on the offer.

186

Now, forty-odd months on it was a different ball game. Gareth, my new boss, was based in Glasgow and fortunately for me had a relaxed approach towards my unusual situation. He seemed happy as long as I delivered my work and wasn't bothered how – or when – it was done.

I knew that my ten years of experience and my excellently skilled – and equally understanding – colleagues were the key. Every day I left the office at 4 p.m., which meant I could collect Steven from school, and thus ensure that Jane was not overtired later. It never ceased to surprise me, on those rare days that it was impossible for me to leave and Jane did have to make the effort to pick him up, how much discomfort she would be in later in the evening.

Naturally there were a few colleagues for whom my early departures caused some resentment. And moving to a new location on the crowded second floor – as we were due to in March – would put my situation even further under a spotlight. Already there'd been comments such as, 'Good of you to come in!', 'Half day again?' and 'It's all right for some' as I packed up to leave. They were generally good-natured remarks and I'd heard them all before but just occasionally, if said in the wrong tone or if I was simply not in the best of moods, it could create an open sore.

'I'd swap a full day for Jane not dying,' I'd once said. It's true to say I was a little concerned at how new colleagues would take to my early departures.

My immediate colleagues, the ones I'd worked with for years and who knew Jane, were protective of me. They would act as my eyes and ears when I was out, letting me know if there were potential problems so I could nip them in the bud.

Mid-morning and everyone had their head down, only the air conditioning's hum could be heard – apart from Darren who was questioning me about the 'Rome to Home' ride.

'What about the phones?' Darren asked.

'Oh, it won't be a problem,' I said.

'You're joking,' he said. 'When Jane's doing an event they go mad.'

I shook my head. 'Not this year, my man. There's no auction, no asking for corporate help and I'm not contacting any national media apart from Sky News and the Press Association.'

Darren looked confused. He pondered this for a few moments, opened his mouth as if to ask a question but decided against it. I put my head back down and made a call.

Minutes later, as I hung up, Darren looked across. 'How are you going to raise any money?'

'I'm not sure. But I guess if Jane inspires people we'll raise the money.'

'But you've said you're going to raise a million.'

'Yeah, I know. But last year's auction was a pain in the arse, it raised five grand and I was like a one-man parcel depot. Plus there was all that aggravation from the people who didn't bid enough. It was a waste of time contacting companies as the vast majority don't want to be associated with Jane.'

'Why?'

'Think about it. Being associated with a woman dying from cancer is not good for the PR image

– it's a PR leper. Individual people we've worked with in the past have moved on and a lot of the taboos have gone but the corporate world is not ready for it.'

Karen, a workmate, arrived with a tray of drinks and placed mine on the desk. 'Cheers, Karen,' I said, taking a sip and moving it to the other side of the laptop.

'I never realised,' said Darren.

I shrugged. 'As much as anything I hate prostituting Jane's death to raise money for charity. So this year, fuck it. A clean shirt with just the website address on and that's it.'

Other colleagues who had started listening in looked round at one another, a little stunned. A silence followed and one by one we slipped the earphones back on and escaped in work.

Toddington services at 10.30 on a Friday morning was quiet, the traffic had been light and we had all arrived early. Luke and I had travelled from Leeds in my car, while Martyn came separately having been filming in the area. We were travelling down to London to discuss with Sky News whether they would cover the bike ride.

Although not strictly necessary for the ride's success, it would give us an indication of whether there would be media interest and whether the sacrifice would be worthwhile.

The event would mean that Jane would spend five weeks away from the family at a time of her life when our natural instincts were to do the opposite. The only motivation to do the ride was to raise money for charity and if either of us felt that wasn't possible, we wouldn't pursue it any further.

I removed my fleece, placing it over the back of the chair only for it to slide perilously close to the floor.

'How's Jane?' Martyn said as he sat down with me at the table.

'Physically she's good,' I said. 'Incredible even – she's planning to do the York Half Marathon in ten days.'

'But, but I thought she only had her last chemo yesterday.'

'She did. And she'll be completely washed out until Monday. Tuesday she'll go back to work. She'll do some small runs in the interim.'

Martyn looked across. 'I'm not very up on these things but I thought the chemo was a strong one.'

'Yes, very toxic. I can't explain how she's managing to do it, no one can. Still she's aware that if she can't do the York Half Marathon now, she won't be fit enough to do the London Marathon and if she can't do London then she won't be able to start the ride two weeks later.'

I'd left Jane in bed, her head raised on two pillows and another one propping her back. A wet towel was draped over the metal bedstead. She'd been up in the night to change her soaking pyjamas and to be sick a couple of times. The chemo had really taken its toll this time. At one point, she had gone downstairs to read as she was unable to get comfortable in bed. And when I got up this morning, I'd wondered whether it was wise to leave her on her own. There was no chance of

190

her coming to London; a round daytrip of five hundred miles was too much to contemplate but she'd insisted I go.

'Is she all right in herself?' asked Martyn.

'She's been quite low,' I admitted.

There was an uncomfortable silence. Depression was something one rarely associated with Jane given her positive public persona and whenever I mentioned to anyone that she was feeling down I could sense their surprise. Although why anyone would think Jane could remain 100 per cent positive 100 per cent of the time remained a mystery to me.

We arrived at Sky News at Isleworth ninety minutes later and Paul and Cassie from the charity SPARKS were already waiting for us. Cassie was the events manager, while Paul dealt with PR and knew Nick Pollard, head of Sky News.

'Nick's just in his office, Mike, we're ready when you are.' Although Martyn knew Nick having done freelance work for Sky as well as last year's documentary, I'd never met him and had only exchanged the occasional email about Jane. Nick though had written a lovely handwritten letter to Jane just before Christmas.

We entered the cramped office one by one. Nick was sitting on a chair to the side of his desk as if trying to create a less formal atmosphere for us and immediately stood up to greet us. We all sat down and Nick immediately asked how Jane was. I said she had been hoping to come down but as she was on chemotherapy it would have taken too much out of her to travel. Nick said how much he'd enjoyed the end-to-end documentary and said he was looking forward to hearing our plans for the next cycle ride in detail.

Jane had created a wish list of events for this year, which at best could be described as fanciful. Bearing in mind her current health, I'd have settled for her being alive in October for the ironman but Jane's list included: York Half Marathon, London Marathon, 'Rome to Home', Salford Triathlon, London Triathlon, UK Half Ironman and finishing with a full ironman in Hawaii.

Already it looked like her hopes of being in the Hawaii Ironman contest had been dashed despite being promised a place. The race authorities were now refusing her entry on the grounds that Jane wouldn't be able to cope with the intense heat. I was a little pissed off about it; there was no opportunity to appeal the decision although I did think if Jane had been American the barrier would not have been raised. We pinned our hopes on the Florida Ironman event instead.

The reason for our meeting today, however, was to concentrate on the ride which would be the year's biggest fundraiser. We hoped that Sky might produce a half-hour documentary at the end of the ride and maybe there would be the occasional news updates. But as the meeting progressed it became clear that Nick had grander plans. There was talk of a satellite van and crew on the road, twice-a-day live broadcasts and a documentary at the end.

We left London delighted. Naturally, there would be compromises and I wasn't sure how

Jane and Luke would react to these. The ride would not be the adventure they had originally planned – it just couldn't be with a full TV crew there. Luke especially had hoped for a sense of remoteness during the ride, a sense of not knowing what the day would bring and cycling for as long as he or Jane wanted with no daily schedule. Inevitably, now that a news crew was going to be following them, that would no longer be possible. The ride would have to have more structure but more money would be raised – and that was the goal all along.

JANE

With assorted maps splayed out on my lap, I sat in the bookstore and studied the scales and distances on each one, checking the annotations and searching through the details. Some scales, I noticed, were too large with too little detail, while others were too small. This would be no good either – it would mean I would have to have dozens and dozens of maps on the whole trip as we'd require six or seven maps per day.

Initially, I looked at road atlases, to give me an idea of the overview of the journey from Rome to Leeds. Should I make my way up to Bologna from Florence or down to Pisa and round the coast? Looking at the routes, the roads through from Bologna were scant and mountainous while the coastal route would mean some death-defying cycling through the narrow blind roads. The sheer drops wouldn't be the thing that killed us, it would be the notorious Italian drivers.

I moved my legs which had cramped up with the uncomfortable position and shifted my rucksack on my back. After several minutes, I gathered up the maps, choosing some for the Italian legs of the journey and placing the French maps back in the metal rotating racks.

Luke and I had come to an agreement that the route decisions were mine, but it was such a vast journey and there were many choices to make. Highlights for me would be cycling through Siena, Monaco and Mont Ventoux. We both said we'd like to go to Paris and this time we would cycle from London up to Leeds through the Peak District.

Back home, there was not enough room at the kitchen table so I spread the maps out on the living-room floor. I unfolded map sheets and shook my head at the immensity of the task. The front door opened and the gust of wind lifted a free sheet. I plonked my pencil case on to it and continued perusing as Mike came in.

'Steven, take your coat off, little man,' he said.

'Dad, Dad, can I put the telly on?' Steven's voice was muffled as he unwrapped himself from his outdoor clothing. He ran through to the living room and picked his way round the maps to turn the television on. The blank screen hissed and crackled with static and remained black for a few seconds before illuminating the dimly lit room.

My solitude and quiet was abruptly ended by the theme tune to the *Power Rangers*. 'Can I get something to eat?' Steven asked. His eyes turning momentarily from the screen.

'Yes,' I said.

'How many biscuits?' he asked, a keen edge to his voice, his blue eyes wide, his face pale below his fluffy tufts that stuck up about his round face.

'Just two, dinner won't be long,' I said.

'What's for dinner?'

'Fish pie.'

'Yummy,' he said with enthusiasm.

Mike stood silhouetted by the hall light through the door. 'How's it going?' he asked.

I lifted my eyes reluctantly from the sheet on which I was tracing a route. 'I can see where I want to go through Italy, but it's just hard work finding the best routes through France. I think if we make our way to Monaco and then down to Nice ... but then it's a huge climb away from the coast.'

'You're still going to climb Mont Ventoux though?' he asked.

'Oh yeah, and before that we'll go through the Grand Canyon du Verdon. It's just the distances I'm struggling with. I've got to go back and figure out where we need to stop. There's one day of ninety-five miles here and that's just too much with the terrain we're going through.' I rubbed my eyes and started to fold up the maps.

'Leave them,' Mike said. 'I want to look where you're going.'

Later that evening I asked Mike, 'Do you think this ride is a good idea? I'm so tired.'

'You'll be fine. You're looking much brighter today.' I did feel a little better. My last session of the current chemotherapy had finished the week before and I was looking forward to getting out on

195

the road for a run the next day. My legs were tight and my head still felt like someone had stuck a mixer through my ear and whirred my brains, scrambling them. Looking at the maps had been hard work as I kept on losing my concentration. One minute a route would be clear, the next I'd be struggling to remember the last town I had circled on the way up through the Continent.

The next day, after Mike and Steven had called their goodbyes from the front door, I dozed in bed. The covers lay heavily on me. My brow was slick with perspiration from my night's uneasy rest. The pillows were heavily indented from my restless turnings. My eyes closed and when I woke again just a few moments later they felt less heavy. I pushed myself from my bed and crept around Mike's strewn clothes, peeping between the curtains to see what sort of day it was. The wind blew light rain against the glass but the sun shone – not the warm yellow light of spring, but a harsher light yellow glinting against a steely grey sky. A crisp packet winged its way up the street, came to a halt and then came blustering back down the hill on the next gust of wind.

Down in the kitchen I munched through some cereal and put some bread into the toaster. Breakfast eaten, I put the painkillers and cod liver oil capsules into the palm of my hand, threw them to the back of my mouth and took a gulp of coffee. I shook my head and gulped, swallowing the lump of tablets, feeling them as they moved down my throat.

Back upstairs, I splashed water over my face and

drew the warm facecloth over my bald head, rubbing my scalp and then patting it dry. I searched through the drawer until I found my lightweight running gloves. My hands were cracked; the chemotherapy had reduced the sensation at the tips of my fingers. Catching sight of my face in the mirror I could still see the effects of the steroids on my eyelids, they were slightly puffy. My cheeks were fuller and flushed. I turned away and headed for the stairs.

Starting at the park gates I headed downhill, letting the muscles in my legs relax. My stride stretching out, I eased myself into the first mile of the run. My head was warm, my cheeks must have been quite pink. The weak winter sun bounced back off the tarmac pavement. I pulled my hat from my head and clutched it in my right hand as I continued over the roundabout heading for the killer hill up to the motorway. The next two miles passed slowly. There were few houses but many cars whizzed by interrupting my concentration. At last I was heading back to Rothwell. I slowed to a walk up the last hill, still feeling the heaviness in my body of the chemotherapy. Reaching the top, I pushed off and resumed running, passing a man well wrapped in his thick grey winter coat, his hat pulled down over his head.

'Keep going, lass,' he said as I drew close to him.

'Good morning.' I smiled as we passed one another.

I could see the corner of the estate and I wanted to slow but pushed myself for the extra yards to make the end of the road. I closed my eyes, hung my arms by my side, my chin dropping down, and sucked in air; the temptation to pant too much, my chest heaved until I gained control over my breathing once more.

Walking slowly back up to the house I stood by the front door and started my stretching routine. Concentrating on each area I went through my upper and lower legs and finally I unlocked the front door and ran a glass of water and sat on the chair in the kitchen. My head dropped and I rested it against the table. The phone rang and my eyes opened.

'Hi.' It was Mike.

'Oh, hello, I've just got in from my run.'

'How far did you go?'

'Six miles. I don't feel too bad. I'm definitely going to run York at the weekend.'

'Oh right. I wished I'd trained a bit harder,' Mike said.

'You'll be fine. I'm going to be slow but I should finish.'

'Good on you. I can't believe it. You've only just finished chemotherapy but you're going to run a half marathon. You really are mad.'

'Oh, don't. I'm not really mad, but if I'm going to get fit for April I've got to start somewhere. Anyway what were you ringing for?'

'I just wanted to check you were okay,' Mike said.

MIKE

Jane's birthday had put me in a quandary. It was her fortieth this year but on the assumption that she'd never reach her fifth decade we'd celebrated in style when she turned thirty-eight. It didn't seem appropriate to repeat the party; especially as a couple of people we were close to and who had been at that party had passed away and their absence would be a reminder of the loss.

Still, the day couldn't pass without some acknowledgement and I'd therefore decided to have a small surprise gathering at home. Suzanne had just arrived from Hull for the weekend and would prepare the house while I took Jane with Steven to Harrogate for the afternoon.

Suzanne sat at the kitchen table working her way through the food like a plague of locusts. She had a baguette grasped in one hand and a lump of cheese in the other. It was a joy to see her teenage angst about her independence had disappeared when she'd left home. Steven came into the kitchen, hair flattened from his bath following football practice, Sunday best on in preparation for the afternoon.

'How was football, Steven?' Suzanne asked, reaching across to give him a hug, but he moved back out of reach. 'Oh,' she said. 'Can't I have a hug?'

'No.'

'Did you win?' she asked.

Steven laughed. 'Don't be silly, practice it was. I don't play in matches, I'm not good enough. Where's Mum?' he asked, sidestepping Suzanne and moving towards me.

'She's still doing her run.'

'She's been ages. She must be running really slowly.'

'It's dinner in five minutes,' I said getting up slowly and creakily – I'd been on a run that morning and the lactic acid build-up had stiffened the joints.

The front door slammed shut as Jane returned home. Coming into the kitchen, she took a swig from the isotonic drink she was carrying and removed the pudding-basin black wool hat which had been covering her almost bald head. Jane looked robust from the steroids, which hid her frailty that was the reality.

'How did you do?' I asked.

'I just can't get a breath going uphill so I'm so slow I'm barely running. I just can't seem to get any strength back. Did you put the water on?' I nodded. 'I'll get in a bath then. Let's set off in an hour. Have you given Steven his dinner?'

'I'm having it in five minutes, I am,' Steven said. Jane smiled and headed off upstairs.

'I'll do Steven's sandwiches, Dad,' Suzanne said, hugging me as she passed. I turned on the radio to drown our voices and we went through Suzanne's jobs for the afternoon: putting up the balloons and banners outside, making sandwiches and snacks, clearing out the living room. 'Do you know what you're doing, Dad?' she asked.

'In what way?'

'A surprise party. What's Mum going to say? She could be furious. I don't want to take the flak.'

'Me neither,' Steven said, studiously avoiding eating the crusts on his sandwiches. 'She's gonna be mad.'

'She's already there, mate,' I said. 'Don't worry

she'll enjoy it and we have to do something. It's a big day we didn't think we'd get to. We need to celebrate.'

I'd carefully considered the consequences of throwing Jane a surprise party and on balance was convinced I'd made the right decision. We didn't have the budget for anything lavish; beer and sandwiches at home were perfect. It was too big a landmark to let it go unmarked, but we needed to avoid anything emotional.

Furthermore, Jane needed a lift. She'd been down since starting chemotherapy in October. That it coincided with her failing health, not being able to train and the dark winter nights hadn't helped, though I suspected the drugs and steroids were a more likely cause of her sombre moods.

Three years ago, we'd worked hard at setting small goals for ourselves: weekends away, rock concerts and nights on the ale. This time we hadn't. I dreaded the rare occasions when Jane would phone me distraught about her prognosis, anguished about what was going to happen. I felt inept at offering any kind of solace and as a consequence she had to look inwards to find a solution; to find peace with herself by coming to terms with the things that made her angry.

It's a strange paradox that the more well known Jane had become, the less time she had to spend with old friends. I'd hoped this evening's party would redress the balance and boost Jane's confidence.

I took Jane and Steve to Harrogate to have tea at Betty's. A treat reserved for special occasions.

I strung the afternoon out as much as I could, delaying our return home so Suzanne had plenty of time, which began to stretch Jane's patience. However, at 5 p.m., as we pulled into our street, the number of cars lining the road was the first indication that anything was afoot.

'Oh,' she said, a smile breaking across her face as she walked into the house.

Inside, there were between thirty and forty people all waiting for the guest of honour. They made the house feel very small. As Jane entered party poppers were pulled and she looked around the room, then went to hug Suzanne, Rebecca, her mum and my mum.

By nine o'clock, most of Jane's siblings who had young family had left while those guests who remained were settling down for an evening of hard drinking. Those balloons not popped were strewn across the floor; streamers and the remnants of the food littered the tables. Suzanne gathered empty beer cans and threw them into a large bin bag that Steve Ridgeway was half-heartedly opening. Jane's jumper was festooned with numerous badges advertising her age. Terry our neighbour looked at Jane and asked, 'Are you all right, love?' He was old enough to be Jane's dad and there was kindness in his voice.

'Yes, it's been a lovely evening. Thanks for coming.'

'Your hair's beginning to come back, Jane,' he said.

'I'll have a grade two in a week or so. Still, I'll have more than Mike soon.'

In the kitchen, several guests congregated,

drinking out of cans.

'Another beer, Terry?' Steve asked as he grabbed a can for himself.

'Don't mind if I do.'

'Tommo?' Steve said handing me a can.

'No, thanks.'

'Bloody lightweight. You're no Paula Radcliffe, drinking's not going to affect your performance.'

'I hope that's the marathon you're referring to,' Mick said.

'Urgh, do we have to?' Suzanne threw a look of complete disgust. We sat drinking and passing the time with the same friends we spent each New Year with; Jane was relaxed and contented.

JANE

Training. There was always training to do. Running before tea some nights. Cycling in the gym other nights after Steven was tucked in. I tried not to let the training get in the way of family life, so Saturday mornings while Mike took Steven to football training were for either long runs or several hours' cycling. Heading out towards York on the bike, struggling up the hills and then heading back towards Leeds and Rothwell.

'Thank goodness, only a short run today,' I said to Mike. It was Saturday morning. Steven was pulling on his shin pads ready for football practice.

'How far are you going? You don't need to do much.'

'No, I'm just doing the six-mile loop today.

Then I've just got to keep myself ticking over.'

'I've looked at my training schedule. Thank goodness we don't have to do this any more after next week.'

'You might not have to, but I do.'

'Oh, yeah. I don't know what you're moaning about, it's only a little cycle ride. I've got to run a marathon. Cycling is easy,' Mike said.

'Yeah, yeah,' I said. 'Anyway you're not the only one running the marathon.'

'Are you sure you should be running?' Mike asked.

'I've bloody well done all the training, of course I'm running. And no, I don't want to run round with you. I couldn't imagine anything worse.'

'I don't want you to run round with me. You'll just slow me down,' Mike said. I raised my eyebrows and gave him a hard stare. Mike raised his arms in a mock submission and mouthed the word 'joke' at me. 'Anyway the sooner you set off, the sooner you'll be back.'

I grabbed my water bottle and turned away from him, stepping into the hall and fastening my watch strap. Heavy rain meant mist and fog swirled round the road, blocking out the sun, making the day feel even colder. I forced myself to start running, ignoring the solid muscles in my leg. I set off slowly, hoping I would feel less wooden as I warmed up a little. The London Marathon was next week and my training had been slow and steady. I felt ready to run the twenty-six miles but it would leave me just two weeks to put together all the final preparations for the real event of the year: the long cycle ride.

A couple of days later, Mike and I had an appointment with Dr Perrin, my oncologist. The news wasn't good. I'd been having regular heart scans while I was on the Herceptin treatment and my last scan had shown a significant drop in my cardiac function. The cardiologist thought my level of fitness meant that I was not incapacitated by this. But maybe that explained why the hills seemed so steep now when I was out running and cycling.

I had to stop the Herceptin and the cardiologist had recommended a treatment called ace inhibitors to help increase my cardiac function.

'Are you still going to run the marathon?' asked Mike as we rushed back to the car after the appointment. It was late. We'd been kept waiting for a long time at the hospital.

'I don't feel ill,' I said, 'so I don't see why I shouldn't.'

'What about the bike ride?'

'Oh, gosh. I don't know,' I replied as we approached the car and Mike pulled out the large bunch of keys. We got in and Mike fumbled with the radio before starting the engine. I sat thinking, watching Mike as he drove.

'We've put so much effort into setting it up,' I said. 'I don't feel any different than I did before Christmas. All that training, all that preparation. I still want to go.'

'Right,' said Mike, not taking his eyes off the road. 'Well in that case, you should go. We should do everything we planned to do. As long as you're sure you want to. You have to decide that.'

205

'I know. And I'm fine, honestly. It'll be a great trip and we should raise a lot of money. Hey, at least I'm here to be able to think about even doing it.'

MIKE

We were caught in the trap of being out on a cold day, five degrees at best, with very few layers on. Walking, limbering up and stretching, we tried not to expend too much energy as we had 26.2 miles to run. Jane was wearing full-length running trousers, knee supports, a long-sleeved T-shirt, a black wool hat and a fetching bin bag to keep in the heat. She was stretching her left calf, thigh and pelvis as they were beginning to cramp up, the result of cold on cancerous bones.

'Are you okay?' I asked, with little enthusiasm for copying her warming up routine. The marathon itself would be sufficient warm-up. There was no need for extra torture.

'I'm cramping,' she said, concentration etched across her face. She grimaced as the muscles tightened. Relaxing the hold after a few seconds, she breathed out and said, 'I'll be all right when we set off.'

When Jane did her last long training run back in Leeds neither of us knew that the Herceptin had given her a chronic heart condition. I was worried that this marathon would put too much strain on it. Mentally I tried to rationalise the fear, after all, nothing had physically changed in Jane, only our knowledge of her symptoms. And

206

although the test results had been summarily dismissed as a polluted test by everyone except Jane, the fact remained that with such results, a patient would usually struggle to climb the stairs. And here was Jane about to run a marathon.

'We don't have to do this,' I said, trying to sound reassuring. Normally I'd have been happy to throw the towel in there and then but I'd trained properly this year and was looking forward to the challenge. It seemed a pointless exercise Jane running the marathon with 'Rome to Home' starting in two weeks' time. Jane's view was that if she couldn't run the marathon she couldn't do the cycle ride.

Jane shook her head. 'I have to really.'

'You don't. No one expects it,' I said.

'Shut up, Mike,' Jane said and turned away.

I paced around before disappearing for a pee behind a tree where I contemplated whether or not to be more forceful in suggesting that she should pull out. Her heart, the leg cramps – this was not the condition in which anyone should start a marathon. But on the other hand, I didn't want to dent Jane's confidence. She was clearly determined to race today whether I said anything or not.

Realising defeat, I remained quiet until we set off. The first mile was two minutes slower than I'd hoped yet Jane kept slipping back off the pace. At the two-mile mark I stopped and waited for her to catch up.

'What are you doing?' she said as she caught up with me. Her cramped-up legs did nothing to help her already ungainly running style. 'You go on. Enjoy the run.'

I could tell I was irritating her.

'Don't spoil your run, Mike. Please go on.'

A wave of guilt overcame me. I knew I should be by Jane's side but at the same time I wanted to run at my own pace. I knew if I stayed with her I'd only irritate her even further and frustrate myself.

'Okay, I'll see you at the finish,' I said and motored off. Through the crowd of runners I picked up pace until I found my natural stride. Motivation for a race like the marathon can come in many different disguises. For the last eight miles on this miserable April day, mine was to finish before a multi-legged caterpillar. Two years previously, it had beaten Jane in the same race – much to mine and Steven's amusement – but this time I'd passed it at mile five as one of the occupants had stopped to take a comfort break.

Turning into the Mall, the finishing line loomed in front of me. The digital clock above it read four hours fifty, so with ten minutes knocked off for getting through the start I was pleased to beat Jane's personal best. But there was little joy at seeing it as I sensed Jane was struggling. Rather than proceed across the line, I stopped a hundred yards short. My run finished I'd wait for Jane and we'd cross the line together.

Ten minutes went by before my body started to cool down and it was only then that I noticed the temperature was perishingly cold. After thirty minutes, I was beginning to shiver, my running shirt was sticking to my skin like a wet flannel to a sink and the exposed leg beneath my shorts was freezing up. I started to question whether it was wise to continue to wait.

I had been waiting forty-five minutes. I tried to figure out the timings but I was so cold it was hard to concentrate. I folded my arms but I couldn't stop them shaking. A spectator who was a fan of Jane's offered me a sandwich and a warm drink which I gladly accepted. I looked up and the grandstand was riddled with raincoats, plastic macs and umbrellas. Heaven really was emptying its bath.

During the next hour, I watched as the race stragglers came in, the grandstand emptied, half the finishing line closed and eventually the public announcer shut up shop. It was with considerable relief that a beleaguered and tearful Jane appeared, hobbling and clearly in intense pain. We hugged.

'You should have called it a day.'

'I'm here now. How long have you been waiting for me.'

'About two and quarter hours.'

'Well, you must be fucking stupid. You should have gone through and got showered and changed.'

'I wanted to wait for you.'

'I despair at you I really do. But, thank you. You must be pleased with your time.'

'Yes, I beat your personal best.' It sounded as if I'd waited for her just to gloat and I was really disappointed with myself for saying it. I discarded the foil blanket I'd been given to keep warm and we walked slowly towards the finish. There were no raised arms in triumph, smiles,

209

waves, joy or sense of relief. Jane described her day to me. How her legs had tightened completely after three miles and she'd failed to reach Tower Bridge in time for her interview with the BBC. She'd decided it was better to finish whatever the time or physical cost as otherwise she'd always regret it. During the last few miles she had occasionally gone into the medical tents to warm up, while outside the course was being packed up.

It was a pointless exercise to everyone except Jane, who knew that whatever circumstances threw at her, she'd find a way of managing. As she finished her recollections, I thought this was surely the end of her athletic year.

By the following Friday the weather had changed and the temperature was 15 degrees higher as I arrived home from work with the sun casting its shadow over the front drive. I dropped my gym bag in the hall and went through to the living room where the patio doors were open and the fragrance of cherry blossom was filling the room. My chest felt slightly heavy, like my lunch hadn't been digested. Steven was seated on a twelve-inch stool, right elbow propped on the low coffee table, left hand holding a yellow crayon. Rebecca was pouring over a pile of photo albums.

'What are you both doing?' I asked.

'I'm drawing a picture of me and Mum, I am,' Steven said, his hand furiously colouring.

'Becca.' I could see at least half a dozen albums stretching across our early married life.

'I've decided to put an album of photos and

pictures together to give Mum for when she goes to Rome. So when she's missing us it'll remind her of how much we love her. Won't it, Steve?'

'Yes it will.'

'Where is Mum by the way?'

'She's gone running, she'll be another thirty minutes, there's a stew on.' I made my excuses and went upstairs to shower and change. When I got back downstairs, Jane was dishing up tea. Any evidence of what Steven and Rebecca had been doing had been cleared away.

There was a melancholy atmosphere as we ate; Jane's imminent departure was hanging over us. When considering whether to do the ride it was never the climbs, mileage or physical strain of the journey which Jane fretted over but the five weeks she'd be away from the family. It's a long time for anyone to be away, but for Jane it could mean a large proportion of the time she had left. As she had been newly diagnosed with a chronic heart condition, we knew there was a risk we might never see her again, and none of us were prepared for that. As we ate, my cheeks began to flush and my forehead perspire.

'Are you okay, Mike?' Jane asked.

'Just a little tired.' I left the table to visit the loo and blow my nose.

When I returned Jane looked at me. 'You sound like you're coming down with a cold. You probably need a few days' rest from training.'

I resented being told that by someone who considered her terminal illness just a minor inconvenience.

'And whose fault is that?' I asked.

211

'I never asked you to wait; that was your own stupidity.'

'Wally,' Rebecca chipped in.

Steven earnestly sat forward. 'What's a wally?'

'Someone who's stupid,' Becca said.

Steven poked at me and said, 'Wally.'

CHAPTER 7

April 2004

JANE

The escalator door slid open and I stepped out on to the upper floor of Terminal 3 of Manchester Airport. Mike, Rebecca and Steven were with me. Mike rolled my suitcase along behind him. My front pannier handle was slung on his back. A white bicycle helmet fastened through its strap banged against his hip.

'Look, there's Luke,' Mike said. I had already spotted him. We had one-way tickets to Rome and Luke was stood guarding our transport back to Leeds. It looked a magnificent steed. Handlebars curled downwards, padded for protection. The back wheel and mechanism was protected by card and board. Everything was taped securely to ensure that even after the baggage handlers had thrown it around it would still be intact for our long cycle ride.

He was dressed in his yellow cycling jacket over

his blue fleece. Long trousers on, to keep out the cold of this chilly April morning. Our older brother Mark stood with him and they both roused themselves as we approached.

'Good morning,' Mark said cheerily.

'Hi. It's a bit early for this, isn't it?' I said.

'You're kidding, we've been here for an hour already. We got some funny looks from the police as well when we were unloading this.' Mark turned and pointed at the bike.

'They looked really jittery,' Luke said. 'Two strange blokes with this huge machine. We didn't hang around too long I can tell you.'

We left Mike and Mark with the children keeping an eye on the bike and we joined the queue to check in for our flight to Heathrow and then onwards to Rome. It was 6 a.m. and my eyes ached with tiredness.

After checking our bags in, Luke and Mark carried the tandem to the outsize baggage area and watched anxiously as the conveyor belt moved forwards. The handlebars caught and the operator leant forward and yanked the bike towards him and then started the belt again. This time the bike slid through with just inches to spare either side.

'Oh, thank goodness,' Luke said. 'I've been having nightmares about that, I just hope it arrives in Rome in one piece now.'

'Well, there's nothing you can do about it now it's gone,' Mark replied. Luke looked pale but he had let out a huge sigh as he watched the bike sent on its way. We moved from the check-in area across the corridor to sit and have a coffee. Mike coughed as he sat hunched in his chair, his shoulders rounding around the ache in his chest. His brow held a veneer of sweat. His fist clenched at his mouth as he coughed again before leaning forward and picking up his cup of coffee.

The clock ticked forward. We still had to go through to the departure lounge and pass through security. Luke and I looked anxiously at each other.

'Last chance to back out now,' Luke said.

'No chance,' I replied.

'Rebecca's got something she wants to give you,' Mike said.

'Oh! What is it?'

I turned towards Rebecca and she scrabbled in her bag and then lifted out a purple-backed book. The textured paper was ornamented with many coloured dots.

'Don't open it now. It's some reminders of what you're missing while you're away,' she said.

'What is it?' I asked again and turned towards Mike.

'It's something Rebecca's been working on for ages. It's nothing to do with me.'

I turned to Rebecca. 'Thank you, it's beautiful. I can't wait to open it.'

I unzipped my bag and crammed the book into the top alongside my medicines and the document pouch with passports and travel and contact information. All the important stuff for the next four weeks through Europe.

Mark stood and hugged Luke and slapped him on the back. 'Good luck,' he said, 'and enjoy it.'

We moved towards the departure area and I

stooped and kissed Steven. Rebecca stood, her arms protectively round herself stiff against my hug and kiss. Mike held me and I put my head against his shoulder.

'Good luck, love,' he said and I lifted my head towards him and kissed him briefly on the lips and then moved away. Walking towards the departure lounge, I held out the boarding pass to allow me through, turning briefly to wave at my family.

The large lounge was crowded with benched seats. Families occupied several of them with their small suitcases and rucksacks strewn around. We made our way to another coffee area and sat in the more comfortable armchairs. I sat a little aside from Luke and slipped off the gold wrapping that held the book closed. The front page had a small message written in blue ink.

To Mum,
Don't forget us when you're having the time of your life. Love, your daughter,
Beccy
X.

By Becca's name was a tiny sticker of a red-pinafored kitten, a tiny sparkling bow over one ear. Inside was a treasure of pictures. Suzanne and me sat on the stairs at our house in Peterborough. My belly heavy with Becca. There were messages from friends and family. Nieces and nephews had drawn me pictures with 'Good lucks'. Steven had drawn a picture of me and Luke on the tandem and signed hugs and kisses after his name. There was a picture of Mike and me in the garden at dusk – a wigwam of beans to the right of us, the sky just reddening as the sun set.

I rubbed my eyes, not wanting to show my tearful emotions. I felt very lonely and scared. I closed the book and wrapped the golden ribbon round it and replaced it in my bag.

As the plane moved towards our final destination, Luke and I looked out of the window. We were travelling over some of the areas we would be cycling through.

'Have you seen that?' Luke asked.

'What?'

'That snow out there.' I looked at the mountains. 'That's going to be interesting cycling that is,' Luke said, his eyes wide with excitement. I felt my cheeks flush with the thought of having to meet the physical demands. I was warm and took off my jacket, I felt energised by the views. The seat-belt sign came on.

'We are now beginning our descent into Rome,' the captain announced. Luke and I craned our necks peering out of the window as the plane taxied to its stand.

Making our way off the plane in our yellow jackets, we walked past the personnel from the plane. 'Good luck, Jane,' one of them said.

'No going back now except on a bike,' said Luke.

'Yeah, that's quite scary,' I said, 'but at least we're on our way home now.'

I was glad I had removed some clothing layers on the plane as the warmth of Rome was a surprise after cool drizzly Manchester. We passed through to the baggage carousel and having retrieved our luggage made our way to the white doors with the sign 'Ritiro Bagagli Fuori Misura'. The English translation read, 'Bulky Baggage Claim'. Luke scratched his head and we both looked around to see if there was anyone to ask for help, not that we could think how to ask. We were just beginning to panic when there was a loud banging from behind the double white doors and our bike was pushed through.

We both bent over, laughing loudly and relieved to have our bike back. We cleared customs and made our way outside. The sun was bright and a woman was walking towards us. She was tanned, wearing tidy shorts and a light-blue short-sleeved top. She looked much cooler than Luke and I felt.

'Jane?' she asked.

'Yes. You must be Sue.' Sue was our contact from the International School in Rome. They had offered to help us with our first steps on our 'Rome to Home' journey by providing a place to stop in for a few days before we set off, and we had gratefully accepted.

'This is Sandra.' She turned and another woman stepped forward. Sandra looked just a little older than me, a woman composed and sure of herself.

'I've got some room at my house so I hope that's okay with you. It's a little way out of the centre but shouldn't take too long to get there.'

'If you wait here,' said Sue, 'Sandra and I will go and get the cars.'

I was starting to feel tired and disorientated. Everything seemed to be moving too fast. Luke and I sat on the kerbside and waited for Sue and Sandra.

'We're here,' Luke said, lifting his face to the sun. 'I don't quite believe it somehow.'

We were hot and tired by the time we reached Sandra's house. My eyes were starting to close and snapped open when the car stopped. I stepped out and was greeted enthusiastically by a dog, who then trotted off leaving me a complete quivering mass. I wasn't just scared of dogs, they terrified me. It was a few moments before my legs started to feel sound beneath my weight.

Luke dragged our bags from the car, and waited for Sandra to advise him where to carry them. Sandra showed him into the house and I stood looking around me, trying to get my bearings.

After her initial greeting, Mara the dog sat quietly in the garden and I had a chance to look around. I could smell the rich scent of jasmine and saw small white stars of flowers climbing over the fence. There were lemon trees and large-leaved hydrangeas. There was an olive tree with its narrow silver leaves.

Sandra had walked back into the garden. 'It's a beautiful garden,' I said and I reached out and pulled a jasmine flower and brought it to my nose.

'Thank you. It's taken a while to get it how I want and it's not quite finished, but I like it,' Sandra said. 'Come on, let's get you inside. I've told my friend Helen we'll meet up for tea.'

We enjoyed a family-orientated dinner at the local trattoria. Sue had brought her children and some of their friends. It made obvious the fact that Luke and I were a long way from our own homes. We said goodbye to Sue and Sandra drove us back to her house. Sandra had made us so welcome, and we were feeling mellow after a glass of wine with our evening meal. Luke had finally unwrapped the tandem and reassured himself it was all in working order.

'How are we going to get that to your hotel?' Sandra asked.

'I've been thinking about that and I think I can use the frame. I packed it in to secure it to your roof rack,' Luke said. 'I hope that's all right with you?'

'Yes, that's absolutely fine. I just hope it works,' Sandra said.

'Oh, believe me, if there's one person I know that can make it work it's Luke.'

The next day, I rose from my bed and stretched the stiffness from my limbs – evidence of our long flight. I dressed for a day's sightseeing in cool loose clothes, and walked woodenly down the stairs. Sandra looked at my face, as I sat down gingerly on a chair at the large table in their kitchen, then looked a little closer.

'Are you all right? You don't look too good.'

'I've not slept much. It's my back I couldn't get comfortable.' I'd spent the night rolling from one edge of the bed to the other, unable to relieve the deep pain in my left lower back. Tears of tiredness and pain eased from my eyes and before I could sweep them away Sandra had spotted them.

'Oh, Jane,' she said softly, taking a step towards me and putting her arms around me. I felt my body relax at the comfort of her touch and the tears fell down my face in a steady stream. 'You don't have to do this,' she said. 'Nobody will

219

think badly of you.'

'I can't give up before I've even started,' I said. 'I just can't. It's taken too much planning.'

'I know all of that, but you don't have to make yourself ill over this you know.'

'I'll be okay. It's just stiffness from the travel I'm sure. When we start cycling properly these pains won't be so bad.'

'Well, we'll all be thinking and praying for you here.'

I smiled at her. 'Thank you.'

'Now let me get you some coffee.'

We finally made it into Rome and found our way to the famous Trevi Fountain. I threw another coin over my shoulder into the fountain behind me. We were in the small Piazza di Trevi, watching the water cascading down the stones through the seahorses of the Neptune chariot. The stone benches that made a semicircle around the fountain were full of people. Many with cameras were crowding to photograph the famous monument. The whole square was milling with people.

There had been much interest in our trip. Our tandem was secured on the edge of the square and I tossed yet another euro coin over my shoulder, smiling for yet another photographer. The painkillers I had swallowed at breakfast had taken the edge from the stiffness and soreness of my back. In any case, it was easier to smile than grimace as we made our way from the square and cycled towards Via della Conciliazione that led to the Piazza San Pietro of the Città del Vaticano where the Basilica di San Pietro stood over the huge square with its semicircle of columns enclosing it. We had reluctantly taken the tandem into the centre of Rome at the request of some of the media, but would not be setting off till the next day.

We strode round the square and then down the long straight road to sit at a café on the pavement, people-watching as we waited for the dark-haired waiter to come and take our order. 'I never thought that we would ever be in Rome thinking about cycling tomorrow,' I said to Luke.

'I know how you feel,' he said. We drank our first cup of Italian coffee and left to make our way back to Sandra's house.

MIKE

'Dad!' Steven's voice rang out from downstairs. I carried on folding the pile of just-washed clothes on the bed but there was an increasing sense of urgency in his voice.

'Dad! Dad!' Throwing the clothes down on the bed so the neat pile I'd formed toppled off on to the floor, I raced out of the bedroom taking the stairs two at a time. In the living room, Steven was sitting in the corner of the couch, his legs straight out in front of him.

'What's up, Steven?'

'Mum was on the telly.'

'When?'

'When I shouted, silly.'

'What was she doing?'

'Riding the tandem with Luke.'

'Is that it?' I said.

He looked at me sheepishly. 'Sorry, Dad. There was some music and Mum riding her bike.'

'Did she say anything?'

'No.'

Steven had not seen his mum for three days. All along the planning stages, we had asked him whether she should go away. His major concern was she would miss his seventh birthday and as a consequence there would be no party. As well as missing Steven's birthday Jane would also be away for Rebecca's GCSEs. But this, we had all agreed, was a good thing as she'd also miss her increasing adolescent mood swings.

Also during the planning stages we had wondered about visiting Jane en route. But, taking everything into consideration, we decided it wasn't such a good idea. For one thing, our family finances wouldn't stretch that far and we figured it might be too disruptive to everyone to just up sticks and head to Europe, where in all likelihood Jane would not be able to spend much time with us anyway as she would have to focus on the ride.

We'd spoken to her occasionally since she'd set off and each time, I'd found the news disturbing. Although we were aware that the travelling would result in a deterioration in her health, we'd not anticipated the extent. My initial reaction was to blame the marathon – but Jane was adamant that it hadn't affected her.

Rebecca had spent most of Sunday cocooned in her bedroom studying. Steven had been patient all day while I'd tackled a number of domestic tasks – mainly the laundry. Jane had kindly left detailed instructions on water temperatures, spin cycles and size of loads.

'Dad, Dad!' Steven's voice boomed out over the opening riff of Guns & Roses 'Sweet Child of Mine' which was blaring out of the television. 'Dad, it's Mum.'

I ran through to the living room just in time to catch the *Sky News* trailer of the ride. My heart sank as I watched her pedal furiously down the road. The house was missing her desperately.

'Thanks, Steve,' I said, grabbing an empty cup and taking it back through to the kitchen where I turned the rings down on the hob and pulled forward the extractor fan hood.

Rebecca bustled into the kitchen. 'Do you know what you're doing?' she asked as she noticed the dryer door popped open.

'Yes,' I said with a sneer. 'Set the table would you? Have you got much revision done?' She didn't respond.

'Dad, can't we have it in the living room? Mum's not here,' said Steven. Here we go, I thought. I had predicted that with Jane away, both Steven and Rebecca would try to test the boundaries but meal times had always been important to us as a family.

'Would Mum let you?' I asked.

'Yes,' he said.

'A likely story,' I said. 'Get to the table.' With only three of us for tea the conversation seemed a little stilted. Halfway through, the phone rang. I got up to answer it.

'Hello?'

'Mike, its Phil Iveson.' Phil was a cameraman

223

for Yorkshire Television. He was in Rome covering the start of the ride. He had been on the John o'Groats ride from start to finish and had become a friend whom we occasionally saw socially.

'How are you?' I said.

'I'm fine.' His South Yorkshire accent made it hard to picture him standing somewhere in the Vatican City. 'I thought I'd give you a call about Jane. She's not well, Mike. We went out to get some preview shots – the snappers wanted them on the tandem – but she could barely get on it.'

'Oh.' My mind began to process what he was saying.

'I didn't know whether to ring. I know there's little you can do about it and even if you were here she probably wouldn't listen to you. But I thought you should know.'

'How bad is she, Phil?' I asked.

'If she's as bad tomorrow I don't think she'll be able to start.'

My insides churned the tea I'd just eaten and I began to feel sick. Breaking the pause, Phil continued, 'Luke's been really good, Mike. We'll all keep an eye out. We were all chatting – Lia, Rob and Martyn – and we're all concerned.'

'Thanks, Phil,' I said and put the phone down. I wandered back to the kitchen were the kids were jabbering away, Rebecca mercilessly teasing her brother.

'Is Mum all right?' Rebecca asked, clearly having caught some of my conversation.

'Yes.'

'That's not how it seemed.'

'She's fine, just a little stiff.'

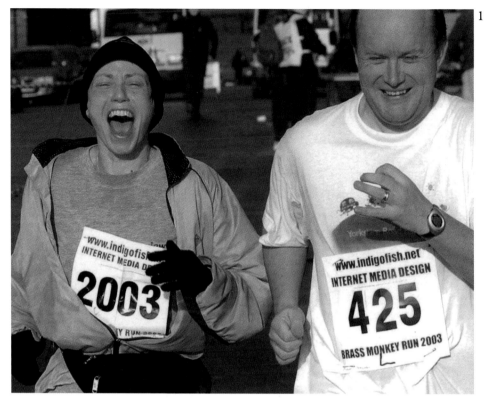

Jane's triumph in the York Brass Monkey Half Marathon in
January 2003 — made harder as she was in the middle of
chemotherapy — confirmed that she was fit enough for her
cycling adventures to begin.

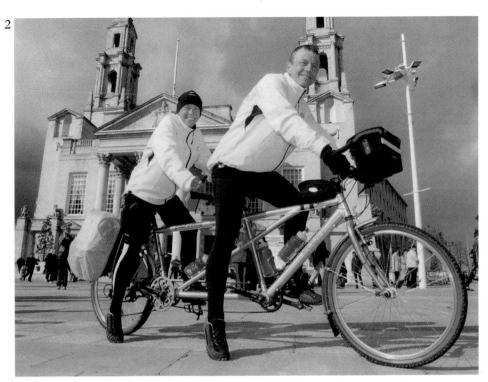

The Cycling siblings, Luke and Jane, pose at the Civic Hall, Leeds on their way from John o'Groats to Land's End.

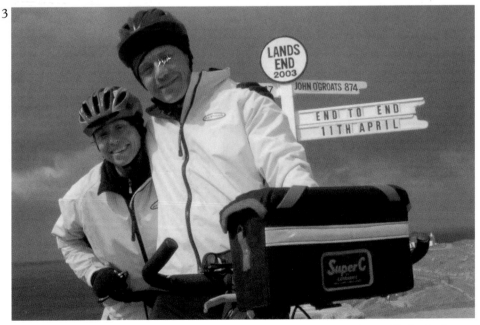

Finally the road had come to an end. Exhausted, at Britain's southernmost point, 11 April 2003.

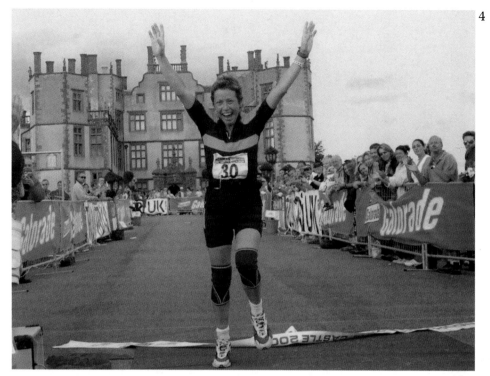

Jane finishing the UK Half Ironman in 2003. Her time of six and a half hours meant that her dream of completing a full ironman might one day become reality.

5

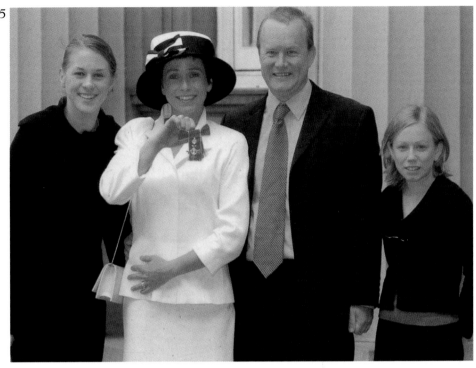

Suzanne, Mike and Rebecca help Jane celebrate her MBE for her services to charity at Buckingham Palace.

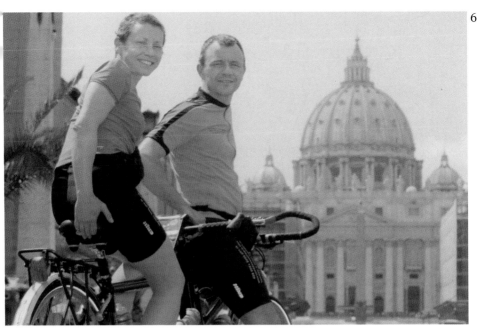

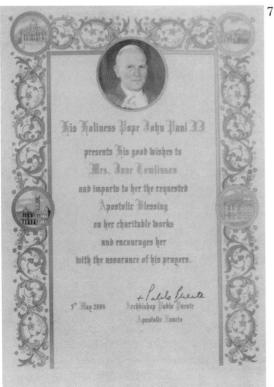

In 2004, Luke and Jane climbing on the tandem once more for an incredible 2000-mile cycle from Rome to home in Leeds, taking with them a blessing from the Pope (below).

His Holiness Pope John Paul II

presents His good wishes to

Mrs. Jane Tomlinson

and imparts to her the requested

Apostolic Blessing

on her charitable works

and encourages her

with the assurance of his prayers.

3rd May 2004   Archbishop Pablo Puente

Apostolic Nuncio

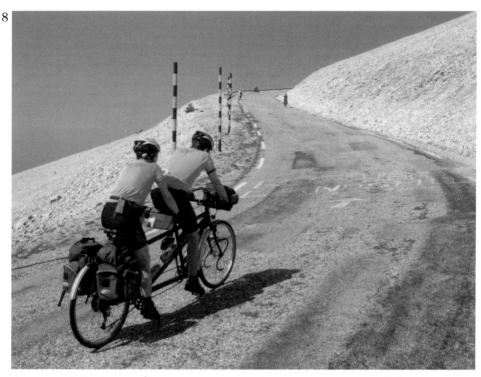

Jane and Luke on the moonscaped upper slopes of Mont Ventoux, one of the Tour de France's hardest climbs.

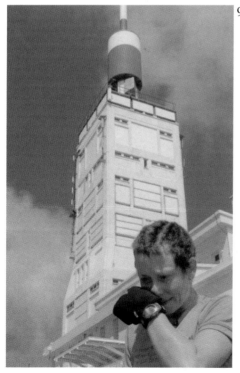

The top of Ventoux — getting there symbolised another year of fulfilled dreams.

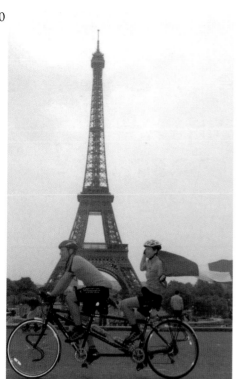

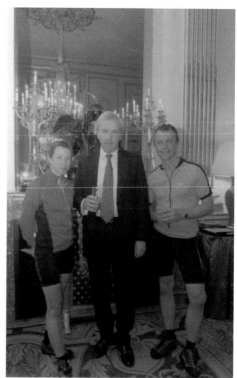

Visiting Paris was one of the highlights of the trip, although Jane and Luke felt that their tandem and cycling clothes struck an odd note at the ambassador's lavish residence!

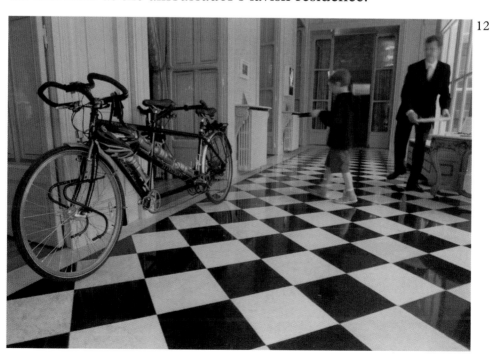

13

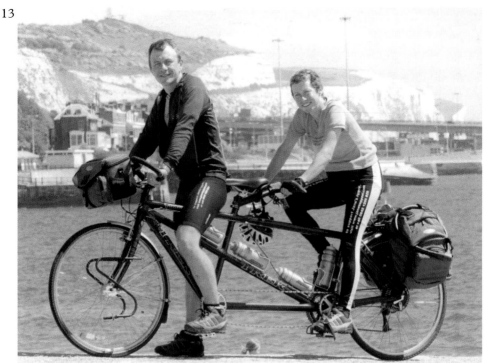

Speeding past the white cliffs of Dover and dreaming of home.

14

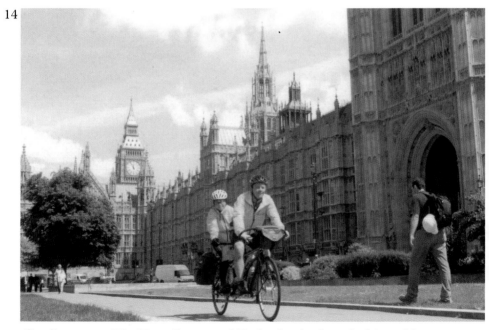

Cycling past Big Ben, Jane and Luke looked as fashionable as ever.

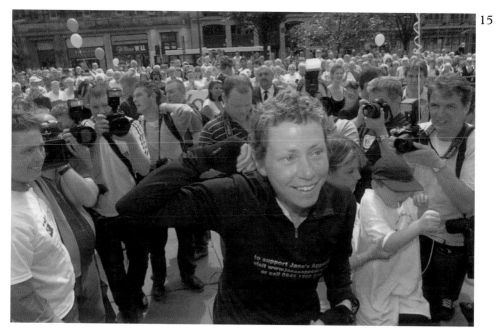

15

Back in Leeds on 7 June 2004, there was an incredible reception.

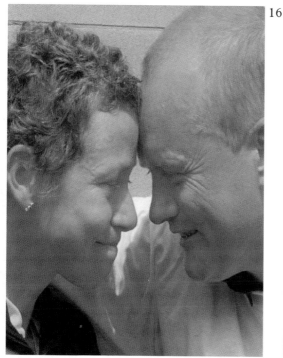

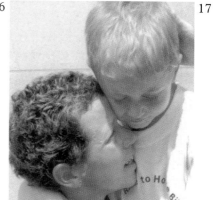

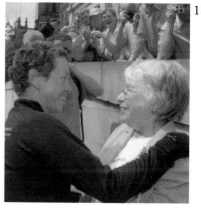

The best bit of all was being reunited with Mike, Steven and Jane's mum.

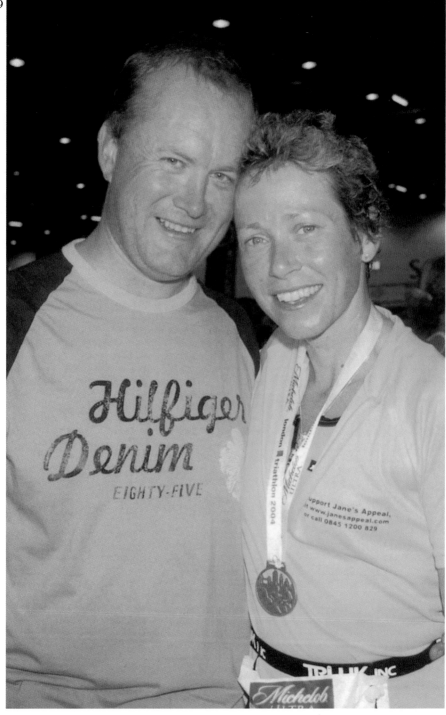

At the London Triathlon later in 2004, Jane — forgetting the agonies of the Rome to Home cycle ride — announced her intention to do a full ironman.

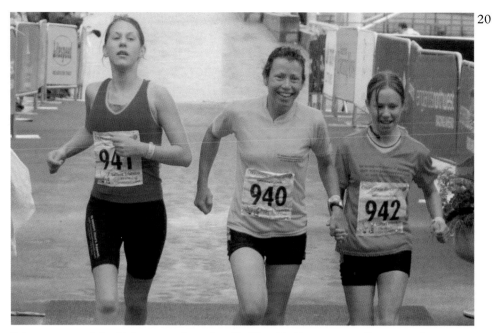

Unseasonable July weather in Salford! Suzanne, Jane and Rebecca finish the triathlon together.

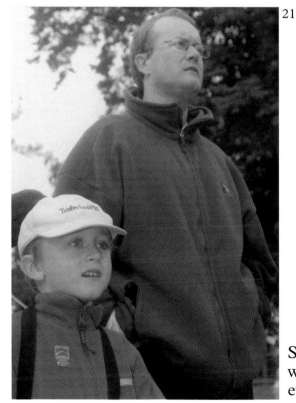

Steven and Mike wondering if they'll ever finish.

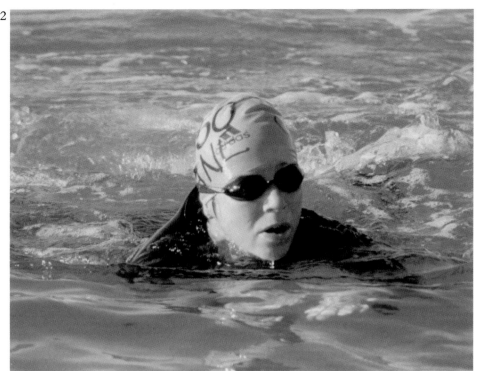

22

The half ironman in Nice was supposed to be a warm-up for the full ironman in Florida but it ended disastrously when Jane was timed out.

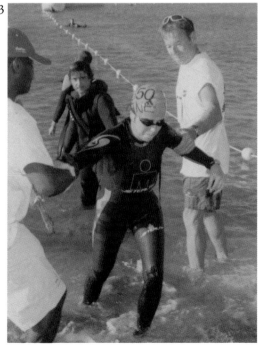

23

Jane's morale plummeted after the Nice triathlon; the swim had been particularly arduous.

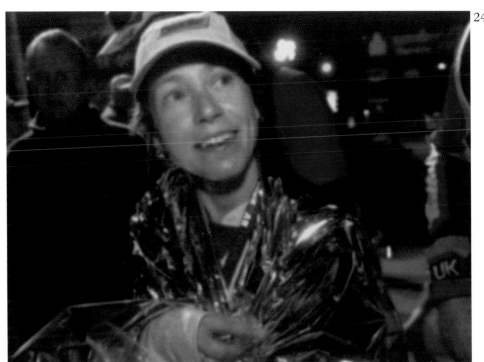

24

In November 2004, overcoming all odds, Jane realised her long-time goal of finishing a full ironman triathlon. Swimming two and a half miles, cycling 112 and running a marathon all in under sixteen hours, Jane was the first terminally ill person ever to complete such an event.

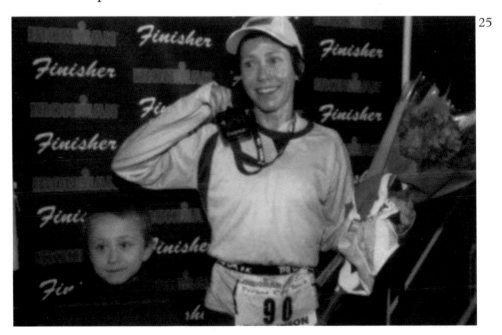

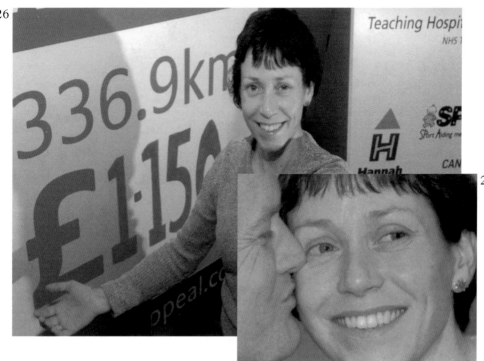

25

In January 2005 Jane announced that she had raised over a million pounds for cancer and children's charities.

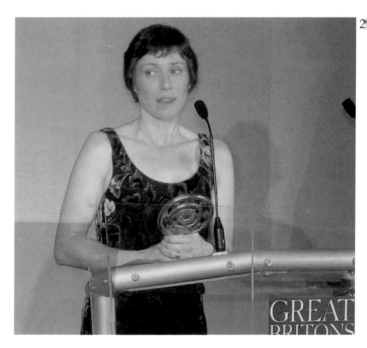

Jane added 'Greatest British Campaigner, 2004' to her collection of awards.

The 3700-mile Ride Across America in the summer of 2006 has been Jane's greatest challenge to date.

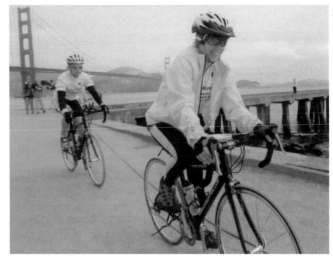

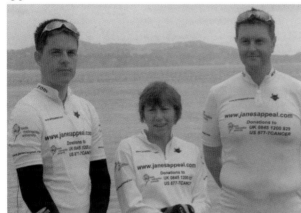

Left of Jane is Accompanying rider Ryan Bowd. On the right is Martyn Hollingworth, the 'cycling cameraman'.

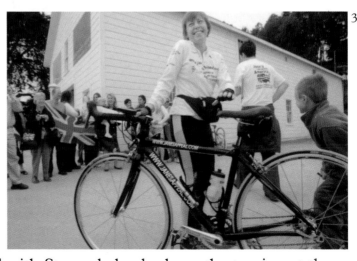

Messing around with Steven helped release the tension at the start of the ride.

Away from the buzz around Jane's fund-raising, the most precious moments are those spent with family.

'Are you sure?'

'Yes. I'll tell you if there's a problem.' Rebecca sensed that I was being economical with the truth but didn't press further.

An hour later, I'd just tucked Steven into bed when the phone rang again. I answered, anticipating Jane.

'Hi, Mike.' Lia's enthusiastic voice took me by surprise. 'I've just put the story out over the wire previewing the ride.'

'Thanks, Lia. Have you had a good day?'

'Busy, everyone had quite a bit of stuff to do so there was a lot of hanging around. You know how it is, people wanting photos of Jane at the Coliseum, St Peter's, Trevi Fountain. Everyone looking for a unique shot.'

'I can imagine.' My eyes followed some kids playing on the road, bikes parked haphazardly on the pavement.

'That's not why I called.'

I had a sense of what was coming. 'Go on.'

'It's Jane,' she said. 'She is very poorly, Mike. I've never seen her this bad. Sky Italia wanted some bike shots and the pain she was in just getting on – you could see it in her face – wincing as her legs straddled the crossbar. She didn't say anything much but she didn't have to.'

I swallowed hard. 'Phil called a little while ago and he said the same thing.'

'Can you persuade her to delay the start?' Lia asked.

'It's not an option,' I said. 'If she can't start tomorrow then we'll have to call the ride off. A delay won't necessarily lead to an improvement in her health. We've just got to hope that things will improve when she starts cycling.'

'What's causing the pain, Mike?'

'Just the extensive amount of cancer, exacerbated by the travel, chemo and the marathon.'

'Oh, Mike,' said Lia. 'Is there anything I can do?'

'Nothing. But thanks for letting me know. I appreciate it and if she gets worse will you give me a ring?'

We spoke for another few minutes. Lia got the odd quote and promised not to report on Jane's fragile health and also to keep me informed. As I lay in bed later I wasn't particularly worried about Jane's health – just anxious that her pride wouldn't stop her from making the right decision. I had spoken to Jane and told her that Phil and Lia had phoned. She corroborated their words and promised not to start if she was too poorly, a promise was that as valuable as a contract signed in pencil.

JANE

Standing outside the hotel, I was shivering in the chill morning air. Ian from *Sky News* who was to be cycling with us and making regular reports to the news programme, wheeled his bike through the hotel door and looked up at the sky.

'Can you tell me, Jane, why we're in Rome and it's colder here than it was when we set off from John o'Groats?'

I smiled. Ian was right. The sun had yet to show

itself and it was decidedly chilly as Martyn, Ian, Luke and I set off on the Via Aurelia to the centre of Rome. The traffic was busy and came close to us as we cycled. In the hour it took us to get to St Peter's Square the sun had burnt away the clouds and the day was starting to feel quite warm. The shadows of the statues of the saints stood out in black relief, dark against the cobbles of the Piazza San Pietro. The cold of the early morning was only a memory.

Luke and I slipped off our tops and sat in the shelter of the columns surrounding the square. St Peter's Basilica in Rome had significance to both Luke and I as Catholics, and had always been where we wanted to start our ride. I unrolled the scroll that I had carried from Leeds. A papal blessing for a safe journey homewards, it would remain in my pannier for the rest of our trip. A dark-haired man on a bike wheeled slowly over to us and nodded.

'So,' he asked in halting English, 'how far as you going?'

'We are cycling to England,' Luke replied.

'Oh, I've just cycled from London.' He bent over his bike and adjusted the straps of his panniers.

'How long did that take?' Luke asked.

'Seven weeks.'

Luke and I looked at one another. 'Oh!' I said.

'We've just got five weeks,' said Luke. The man looked at us and then at our bike.

'Good luck, I think,' he said, mounting his saddle and sliding from view.

A small crowd had gathered at the front of the

square. A group of young adults stood alongside a banner from the British International School which said 'GOOD LUCK, JANE'. A couple of the students held other banners – one in the green, white and red of the Italian flag had the words 'ROME TO HOME' written on it alongside a wonderful picture of a bicycle. Another said, 'GO JANE GO'.

'Thank you for coming out to support us today,' I said to the smiling faces who had gathered in the square. 'The whole trip is quite daunting.'

'Which way are you headed out of Rome?' one of the parents asked Luke.

'Well, I rely on the navigation coming from the back of the bike,' Luke said, nodding his head in my direction. 'In fact, the first time I know about the route is when I'm given directions from the back.'

I looked at my watch. Ian stood waiting by the camera crew. *Sky News* was covering the start live. The time had been set for 9 a.m. British time, 10 a.m. our time.

'Is it time to go?' Luke asked. I nodded and so he stepped over to the shade and he wheeled the bike out towards me. I felt relieved to be finally setting off, after all the planning at last we would be turning the pedals heading homewards.

Sitting astride the bike, we pushed down and set off a little unsteadily at first. I turned in my saddle, ignoring the pain in my back, and waved at the people who had come to send us off. My glasses in my hand, I pushed them on to my face and, with one last look back, turned towards the direction we were travelling. We were off.

We coasted round the corner of a red brick building and turned right again away from the square and towards the centre of Rome. Cars roared by us, beeping their horns, braking suddenly as they pulled around us but still leaving us plenty of room. I felt excited that we were finally on our way, the busy foreign roads only added to that excitement.

After half an hour we passed over the River Tiber at Ponte Cavour and then made our way to Via Flaminia, which would take us back over the Tiber and up and out of Rome. When we approached the Ponte Milvio, a white bridge, we could see a set of traffic lights.

'We need to move across to the left,' I said. Glancing behind me, remembering a conversation with Sandra about Italians and exaggeration, I put out my left arm and made a gesture as big as I possibly could.

It worked. The cars flashed their headlights and beeped their horns but they held back, allowing us a smooth passage through the labyrinth of vehicles and red brake lights. We came to the bridge and stopped, having to lift the bike over a chain set across the bridge. A man stood there, his guitar held out in front of him, plucking at the strings.

After the bridge, we toiled up a long hill through the outskirts of Rome. The cadence of our pedalling fell and we moved slowly, our bodies rocking from side to side to maintain our momentum. Cars passed to the left of us and we kept to the kerbside. Some roared past, without even a glance from their drivers. Others slowed down to take a good hard look.

One car pulled alongside us, indicating the next right turn ahead. We pushed on but the woman driver zoomed across us, causing Luke and me to brake so that we didn't hurtle into the side of her car. She wound her window down and shouted unintelligible Italian at us.

'What?' yelled Luke, frustrated, as she shouted something at him leaning from her car. 'Oh, go away.'

I leant round the bike and shouted back, waving my arms at her. 'Hey. Get outta of our way, woman.' Startled, she drew herself back into the car and sped off away from us.

'What did you say to her?' asked Luke, clearly impressed.

'I've no idea,' I replied. 'I just did what Sandra said and talked loudly with my hands like the Romans do.'

We set off again and, two hours later, we finally reached the end of the climb and sped along quieter roads to Lago di Bracciano. We could see the castellated town of Bracciano to our right. It was early afternoon so we detoured from our route, following the signs for 'Il Centro' to find somewhere to eat.

We chose sandwiches from the local café and pushed the cycle to a small piazza. The sun was high in the sky and bounced off the white fountain that dominated the square.

'This beats the bench outside that small town in the Dales,' Luke said as I brushed crumbs from my chin.

'That was Leyburn, wasn't it?' I said.

'Yes, and it's not raining. Do you want an ice cream?'

I nodded. 'I'll get them,' I told him, crossing the street to drool over the *gelato* selections, returning with sugared cones, two scoops in each. The sun was already melting the soft creamy ices.

'I hope this is the first of many,' I said.

The roads were quiet; the cars that did pass hooted their horns to warn us of their approach before skirting us widely. As we neared Lago di Vico the sun was clouding over but we were still grateful for the shade of the trees above the lake as we started to climb long hills towards our evening's destination.

'Do you want to stop?' Luke called over his shoulder as we panted up a short hill. Sweat was trickling down his neck.

'I'm all right,' I called back.

The sun had disappeared completely by the time we made the last long climb into Viterbo, a small town roughly fifty miles north-west of Rome. Small drops of rain splashed on to our bare arms. The rain shower made the roads greasy and as we set off at a set of traffic lights the front wheel slipped to the right sending the back wheel out and us crashing to the ground. I sat on the tarmac making sure it was just my pride injured. We arrived at our hotel, tired and hot and fed up.

'I thought we were having an easy first day,' Luke said, standing over the upended bike fine-tuning the gears and checking the brakes.

'It was the late start. It's too hot to cycle in the

231

middle of the day,' I said. 'It was a lot hillier than I thought as well.'

'How far did we come?' Luke asked.

'Fifty-four miles and we climbed just over six thousand feet.'

'Easy day, my foot,' Luke said and turned his attention back to the bike.

Learning our lesson from yesterday, we rose earlier than we had planned and had fourteen of the sixty-five miles out of the way before 9 a.m. The weather had changed to drizzle with periodic heavy showers. So frequent and short were the showers you almost forgot them once they were over and our speed on the bike meant we dried out quickly.

Stopping for breakfast at the small town of Marta, we sat by the shores of Lago di Bolsena enjoying booty from the hotel's buffet: croissants and small chocolate cakes. I turned my back on the grey rippling water and looked at the old stone houses just yards away. A small round woman stood in her window looking out. Her hair was covered by a black shawl but grey wisps showed at her temples; her brown hands stroked a comfortable ginger cat.

I brought my water bottle to my lips. Now my stomach was full I could take some anti-inflammatory tablets.

'How's your back?' asked Luke.

'It's not as bad as yesterday. I think the cycling has stretched some of the spasm out of it.'

'That's good.'

We replaced our water bottles in the cradles

and secured the panniers, hooking the yellow waterproofs over them to protect them from the showers. I shrugged my shoulders back, stretching my neck and preparing myself for another few miles hunched over the handlebars.

We climbed up and out of Marta and then continued up along a steep climb through a mountain pass. The road was a smooth black stripe and the bike sped along. We could hear the bells hung around the necks of goats in the grassy hills to our right. A resounding clang that echoed musically around the hills. The rain started once more and looking behind me I could see an arc of water reaching more than two bike lengths behind.

'At least we know our mudguards work,' chortled Luke.

The rain continued as we pushed our bike under the veranda of our hotel on the outskirts of the city. We looked out over the long snaking climb we had just finished.

'It's like a postcard,' Luke said, pointing down below the city walls of Pienza to where we could see the road switching back on itself. The rolling plain below stretching into the distance was punctuated with tall cypress trees that made green exclamation marks all the way into the distance.

'It's not far to Siena.'

'Is that where we're headed for?'

'Yes, it's just over thirty miles,' I said. 'A short day to give us time to look round the city. You'll love Siena it's got a beautiful square.'

It was a tough couple of hours cycling and, as we neared the ancient walled city, the rain which had wetted us all morning turned heavier till we could hardly see through the dense curtain of water. We pushed the bike into the main square, the Piazza del Campo, famous for the horse race where bare-backed riders speed around the cobbles. Taking it slowly down the steep lane, the cobbles slick with water, the rain dripped from our helmets on to our faces, down our necks. Water ran down the small of my back as we searched for somewhere to secure the bike.

'I imagined sitting here sunning ourselves enjoying *gelato*,' I said to Luke as we shivered over cups of sweet chocolate drinks watching the rain. We were still cold as we made our way from the shell-shaped Campo out of Siena to our hotel.

That evening, Luke ventured back into Siena to eat. I sat alone in the hotel, eating some pasta and watching the procession of ants crawling through the baskets of fruit and bread on the table next to me.

Breakfast was laid out the next morning on the same table that the columns of ants had marched over the evening before. The thought of it stopped me from picking at the bread and cheeses. I drank milky coffee, spooning some extra sugar into it to keep me going. It was another short day in miles, but the climbs through the Chianti region would be challenging on our heavy bike.

The storms of the previous day were almost just a memory. There was just the odd puddle of water steaming in the sun, which even at this early hour was radiating warmth on to our bodies. From outside I could hear Italian voices and turned to see Luke talking to a group of older men. One bent double had on a dark hat and was talking earnestly to Luke, who was struggling to understand what he was saying.

The man was circling one leg and pointing to Luke and then me and then back to the bike.

'Si,' Luke said. 'A Londra tre mila chilometri.' The old man nodded and turned to his compatriot speaking rapidly. They all turned and smiled.

'Molte béne,' he said. 'How do you say?' His eyes lifted as he tried to think of the words. He raised his hands in a small questioning gesture. 'Ah. Bon voyage. Good luck, I think,' he said and reached across to Luke and held him by the shoulders and kissed both cheeks. He reached for me and I was greeted in the same way.

'Grazie,' I said. Luke wheeled the bike over and we mounted it and set off to a rousing cheer from the Italian tourists.

The hills were steeper than the previous day. We travelled through a jewelled patchwork, the acidic green of the vines contrasting against the soft smoky green of the stunted olive trees. The map showed the road wriggling through Chianti. The more bends and turns on paper, the steeper the gradient when cycled as the road climbed and climbed through the rolling hills. We passed many small towns, tall churches with square naves and pink-stoned castles. The respites on the downhills were sweet but never lasted long before we had to push ourselves up and over another hill.

Other cyclists on the road would lift their hands

and greet us with a quick 'Ciao' that seemed to disappear in their mouths as they called it. Luke, catching sight of a multicoloured cycling vest in front, pushed forward, eager to catch the unaware traveller. We ate up the distance between us, our bike singing and thrumming against the road. Wheels hissed against the tarmac surface till we were on the shoulder of the slim athletic cyclist, who turned and looked at us, bewildered at the beast that was passing him by. We lifted our hands in unison and called 'Ciao' over our shoulders and carried on down the road. I looked back and could see the man collecting himself as he took a sip from his water bottle.

'I think he's going to try and come back after us,' I called to Luke.

'That's what he thinks. Come on, let's give it some welly.' We turned our legs faster and I glanced once more over my shoulder to see the cyclist fade away behind us and then stop by the roadside.

Cycling towards Florence from the south we were high above the city and could see the red brick of the Duomo and the stretch of the Ponte Vecchio over the River Arno. We dropped down rapidly to the city and reached the banks of the river which moved a rapid swollen brown mass under the bridges. We crossed the river and the brief sunshine we had enjoyed disappeared as we struggled to push our bike along the busy Street outside the Uffizi.

Cars beeped at us as we stepped out into the street to avoid knocking the legs of pedestrians.

236

We tried to make our way to the Ponte Vecchio but the rain poured from the sky and we were struggling too much with the bike so we gave up and cycled out towards our hotel.

The Firenze Hotel was a rambling old building but it had a comfortable lounge with inviting armchairs and a large room for us to share, which we draped with our newly washed damp clothes. The sky turned blue once more and we walked into the city centre to climb the 463 steps to the top of the Duomo. Admiring the beautiful white, green and pink marble, we walked around the painted ceiling depicting the Last Judgement by Vasari and Zuccaro. Panting our way to the top we were rewarded by views out over the city.

'That's where we came in,' Luke said, lifting his finger and pointing far into the distance.

We met up with the British Consulate, Moira McFarlane, who had contacted us after reading about our ride. She took us high above the city to the Giardino di Boboli and pointed to a group of buildings.

'See that,' she said, 'that's the Palazzo Pitti. Back in the sixteenth century the Medici family had Vasari's passage built.' She rolled her Rs in a rich rumbling Scottish way quite different from the sharp rolling of the Italians. 'It meant the family could walk to the Uffizi without having to move through the noise and stink of the Ponte Vecchio.' The bridge she was referring to stood gleaming yellow in the late sunshine; three open arches covered with buildings.

Luke and I ate out at a family restaurant nearby. 'How's Karen?' I asked him.

'Oh, she's okay. She's decorating the house to keep herself busy. What about Mike?'

'He still sounds really poorly, he's going back to the doctor's later this week. I'm sure he'll be fine.' We sat in silence thinking about our own families.

It was a busy and frustrating morning cycling out of Florence. The traffic buzzed by us and the cars cut in front. We were glad when the roads became a little quieter as we headed west towards Empoli. We followed the river swollen with the previous day's heavy showers, the banks were flooding, trees submerged to the lower branches. We bent low over the handlebars and ground out mile after mile on the flat dull highway that lead us towards Pisa. It was slow going, and late afternoon by the time we reached Pisa. We still had an hour's cycling to reach our evening destination – the ancient Roman outpost of Lucca. Standing in front of the famous leaning tower we felt no joy at being there.

'Just our luck to get a headwind on the first flat day,' Luke said.

I nodded. 'It's just so draining,' I said quietly. 'The wind is against you all the time. I'm so tired.'

'At least we are moving into quieter roads – that traffic into Pisa was awful.'

We got back on the tandem and set off towards Lucca. Moving northwards we were no longer cycling directly into the wind and some gusts helped thrust us onwards towards our evening destination. We circled the tall red-brick city walls that gave the appearance of a military outpost to the quiet city hidden within.

'Shall we cycle through there in the morning?' I said.

'I think so, its time to get done for the day,' replied Luke. A day of sunshine and showers ended abruptly with a heavy downpour soaking us to the skin before we could reach our digs for the night.

It was well worth the effort returning to the city centre the next day. We made our way to the central square, the Piazza del Mercato. It was an oval-shaped piazza, originally the Anfiteatro Romano, now enclosed by ancient houses. It was early morning and the open space was empty as we cycled round and round the ramshackle buildings with red-tiled roofs. Pigeons whirled in the air, flapping their wings, as they gathered around a bearded man scattering bread for them. We exited through the narrow alley and headed out of the city towards the coast at Viareggio.

We entered the marina and cycled over several small canals before we finally had to admit we were lost; we had strayed from the main road.

'Il centro?' I asked a man who was looking at us. 'Ah, si,' he said and pointed back where we had come from.

We carried on cycling forward, past large groups of cyclists clad in multicoloured kit, with light road bikes. Luke watched as they sped past. 'The next group that comes by – I want to stay with them,' he called. Moments later, a large group was approaching us from behind and Luke upped the tempo of the bike. As the group came alongside they waved their hands. The leader called 'Ciao' and cycled ahead of us but we had had time to make their pace and we caught the end of the group, speeding alongside the dozen or so cyclists. One by one they turned and looked at us. The heavy tandem, the dark panniers, our touring clothes, our legs circling rapidly as we drifted within the group. Luke started braking to keep us alongside as we began to carry through the group. We slowed as we neared the traffic lights that had turned red, but watched as the cyclists skipped the lights and sped off.

'What do you reckon?' Luke asked.

'Stay with them.' We speeded up and, watching the traffic to the right, headed through the red light till we caught the group again. For half an hour we enjoyed their company until they turned off and we continued on up towards Massa.

'That was fantastic,' Luke called as we settled into a quieter rhythm. 'I've just met one of my life-long dreams of cycling in a peloton.'

La Spezia was a busy port town and our meagre hotel was on the outskirts in quite an industrial area. We walked into the city centre and sat on the prom looking out over the sea. A large group of old Italian men stood enjoying the sights and singing deep throaty songs. We had attracted their attention and I heard the word *straniero* meaning foreigner. One turned to us and asked, 'Di dove sei?'

'Inghiltera,' Luke replied and soon he was standing with one of the old man's arms around him, a glass held forth as we became just briefly one of their group. As they made their way back on to the coach they'd arrived in, a grey-haired man held back and from his cavernous checked bag produced a bottle of homemade wine.

'Grazie,' Luke said and we received a largely toothless grin in a polished brown face.

The roads were meandering into and out of the coast. The main route was too busy for bikes so we headed inland through the foothills of the Apennines.

'I want to know why we have to start each day with one of these big long climbs,' Luke said from the front of the bike.

It was a slow start to the day and we climbed steadily, passing through three long tunnels. Cars buzzed past us, their echo staying long after the tail-lights had disappeared.

'Look at that,' I said and swivelled in the saddle to look back at the pink house with the painted grand façade. We past more and more of these magnificent trompe l'œil buildings on our way into Varese. Motorbikes roared past us and we could hear them chopping their gears as they turned the corner and hit the steep ascent up to the Passo di Cento Croci.

'I think we need to get something to eat before we go any further,' I said to Luke as we entered the main piazza and sighted a likely looking café. We ate enormous toasted cheese and ham sandwiches, washed down with freshly made milky coffee. Donning our helmets once more we headed out of the town.

241

'What do you think?' I asked Luke as we saw the road ahead of us twisting and turning high up into the dark-green ridged hill.

'What do I think?' he replied. 'I think this is a bit soon after dinner.' We put our heads down and edged the bike up. A leather-clad motorcyclist roared past us, then another and another, making Luke steer close to the edge of the road. Each corner we came to was a blind bend climbing steeply up and up. Sheer drops on the side with only a small crash barrier up to the top of our thighs. Our bike slowed, but the small gear allowed us to circle our legs and slowly creep up the hillside. At last we passed the blue sign showing us that we had reached the summit. We pulled over and sat on the grass.

'What's that?' Luke asked pointing at the package I had pulled from the pocket of the pannier. Inside a clear, white-spotted, crinkly plastic package was the remainder of my dinner from the hotel.

'It's pizza from last night.'

'I know that but what have you kept it in?' I lifted it up and took out an enormous slice. 'Oh, that's a shower cap. There wasn't anything else to put it in.' Luke bent over double, laughing at the sight. 'Do you want some?' I stretched out the package to him.

'No, thanks, I'll stick to my dried fruit and nuts.'

Another monstrous pass saw us strewn roadside once more, panting, our legs shaking with the effort. We looked ahead and could see dark hills, dwarfed and stunted trees silhouetted against the low sun; the day was drawing to a close. In the distance was a large peak, patches of snow white against black.

Our hands clung to the handlebars, chilled, our heads hung low, our legs circled round and round. The road disappeared round another bend.

'Oh, no. Can you see where the road goes now?' Luke asked, pointing ahead. We could see the road rising above us in layers. The green below us was a stark contrast to the grey earth and dark brown winter-stained trees, still to erupt in bud. The small towns we had passed were distant little models. Houses were bright squares topped with red triangles. As we cycled higher, the air chilled, the trees were still bare of leaves and snow lay in drifts by the side of the road. Our breath was a brief mist as we exhaled and inhaled deeply, our lungs bursting. The small patches of snow became one mass from which erupted dark grey hillside. We had known we had a climb but hadn't realised just how tough it would be.

'How much further is it now?' Luke asked as we stopped at the side of the road and stood astride the bike while we shovelled food in our mouths.

Legs shaking from the exertion, I wiped the damp from the GPS navigation system and looked at the route. 'We've just got one more switchback to do and then we're at the top.'

'It just keeps going and going,' Luke said. We rounded one last corner and caught sight of the welcome blue sign Passo del Tomarlo. 'How high are we now?' Luke asked.

'Just over four thousand eight hundred feet.' We

crested the hill and swooped down it. 'That's better,' I said as the strain was released from our legs and the bike rolled down the hill of its own volition like a spring released using all the energy we'd put into it on the way up.

Luke was shivering with cold when we entered the quiet ski resort of Santo Stefano d'Aveto. 'I wish you had let me put on a top before we set off down.'

'Well, at least we're here now.' I pulled out the last piece of my pizza from my shower cap and bit into it as the hotel manager brought over hot drinks. Luke was filling his face with a large piece of bread, still attempting to take away the hunger pangs that had struck him on the hill.

'See, it's not always uphill,' I shouted from the back, as we swept along the next morning. Luke shook his head and raised his shoulders in disbelief.

'You'll be telling me this is a flat stage next,' he said. The road was smooth and the bends were sweeping enough for us to keep a good speed up as we made our way down. We could make out silver ribbons falling down the side of the passes. Huge thundering waterfalls, silent in the distance. We started to pass signs for the Giro d'Italia and frantically tried to find others that would indicate where the cyclists would be coming through. The Giro is the annual professional cycling race round Italy.

'Look,' I said to Luke. 'Boasi, that's not far from here.' We raced up the narrow steep road towards the hill-top town. The advance caravan of cars and other supporting vehicles passed us on their way down. There was a pink car with a grey squirrel on the top, and loud music and blaring voices. They all beeped as they passed and we raised our arms. Luke put out his hand to stop one of the official merchandise cars.

Handing over his five euro note he was passed a bag. 'It's like a birthday, isn't?' he said, peering in and pulling out a soft toy. 'It looks like a mad squirrel.' In fact the small grey toy clad in a pink T-shirt was quite cute. Luke pulled on the pink T-shirt and set his pink cap on his head. 'Do you think I could get a job dressed like this?'

'Well it's quite fetching. I'll give it that,' I said. We made it before the bikes passed through and stood waiting just below the tunnel at Boasi. Activity seemed to increase and a man placed himself in the centre of the road with a red flag just as the team cars sped through. There were crowds of people all stood at the roadside craning to see as the official motorbike passed by. Then the cyclists were upon us, they passed just inches from us, reaching speeds we could only dream of on our bike.

'Wow,' I said, my mouth dropping open in sheer astonishment at the spectacle of so many cyclists massed together. Forming a huge peloton, they streamed past us too quickly to be able to sight where the current leader in the Maglia Rosa, pink jersey, was.

'We'd better put our foot down,' Luke said 'We've still got to get past Genoa and I promised I'd get you to our hotel by five.'

'We'll manage,' I said. 'Besides it was worth the

side trip.'

As we journeyed through Genoa, the sun was high and the streets heavy with traffic. Back on the busy coastal road the tour buses, cars and lorries swept wide by us, leaving us in our narrow metre stuck alongside the wall of the cliffside. Luke wore his pink Giro T-shirt proudly as we continued on towards Arenzano.

In Arenzano I stood jigging around trying to keep warm as the engineer from Sky set up his equipment ready for a live interview with the studio.

'It's a good job I've got a jumper on,' I said, the warm day was turning to a brisk cool evening.

Rob, the producer, called out, 'Can you look down here, Jane?' He turned a small monitor towards me and on the screen outlined against our lobster-red walls were Rebecca, Steven and Mike. I was surprised to see them on the screen. They were all smiling at me and then looking down at a monitor to see me.

'Hi, Steven,' I said. 'Have you had a good birthday?'

'Yes,' he replied quietly.

'It's good to see you all, you're looking really well.'

'So are you,' Rebecca said.

'We know that,' Mike said. 'We see her every night, don't we, Steven?'

Steven nodded. The link stayed open for over five minutes then Rob tapped me on the shoulder. 'We have to finish now, Jane. I'm really sorry,' he said.

'That's okay,' I said, as he unhooked my microphone and ear piece and handed them back to Neil the camera guy. 'Thanks everyone, that was amazing.'

The tears I'd tried not to show my family were close now and I stepped away from the camera crew and walked to a small benched area nearby where they flowed and my sobs came tearing from my throat. An old man came over and looked at me, raising his eyes quizzically and speaking rapidly at me. I just made out the words 'Male mi dispiace.'

I looked at him, confused. 'Non capisco, Inglese,' I said, the words catching in my throat with the sobs, and he held his hand out and wiped away a tear from my cheek. Weakly I returned his smile and brushed the tears away.

'E non c'e male,' he said looking at me.

I nodded. 'Si non c'e male, grazie.' He lifted his hands to his shoulder in an open gesture, 'Prego,' he said and walked away.

MIKE

My eyes stung, flickering involuntarily. I took a swig of water from the plastic cup. As Jane's trip had progressed, so the housework had started piling up, meaning I was often working into the early hours of the morning.

Today we'd risen early because it was Steven's birthday. He'd bundled through on to my bed, shouting for Rebecca to join him; she'd already been up for an hour straightening her hair and choosing her day's wardrobe. Jane's absence was keenly felt by all three of us, the empty space next to me in bed an all too physical reminder.

We knew it wouldn't be the same without her but, at the same time, Rebecca and I ensured it wasn't a sad occasion. Steven at least did have the solace of knowing that he had his official birthday 'like the Queen' to come when Jane returned home; two lots of presents appeases any seven-year-old.

In the afternoons at work, I found myself getting increasingly anxious as the hours wore on, waiting for the call from Jane confirming that she'd finished the day's ride. Once she'd phoned, whether it was at work or home, there was huge relief.

Sunday had been particularly tense, waiting for Jane to finish at Santo Stefano d'Aveto. It was thought that they'd get there by one but they didn't arrive till just before six. A lack of communication exacerbated the situation. Rob from Sky had given me regular updates as to what was happening but because of the high altitude and remoteness, it meant that reception was poor and that would leave long gaps in the afternoon where we had little – or no – information. Knowing that they were cycling through the snow line, together with comments such as, 'We must have taken the wrong turn as they can't be cycling up here', was little comfort.

Today I worked silently, my only interruption the occasional phone call. I knew I'd be likely to snap at colleagues, barking out orders irrationally as the afternoon progressed. My stomach felt as though an army of cross-stitchers were working away in there; the palms of my hands sweated, fingers stuck to each other.

At just after three my phone rang. I lifted the receiver immediately, 'Hello.'

'Hi Mike.' It was a familiar female voice from the BBC, though I struggled to find the name it belonged to. My mind flicked, it'll come to me.

'How's Jane?' she asked.

'Okay,' I said. 'It's been a tough day of cycling but they are still in one piece.'

'Are you going over to France at all?' she asked.

'Yes, Sunday, to watch Jane climb Mont Ventoux on Monday.'

'Mmmm,' said the voice. There was a moment's hesitation, as if she was contemplating whether or not to ask her next question. 'You don't have to, but we wondered whether you would do an interview with us before the weekend?'

There was just something about the way she phrased it, the tone of her voice that made me slightly alarmed. 'What's it for?' I asked. 'Anything in particular?'

'It's er ... erm, it's er ... not for use straight away,' she said. The penny dropped. 'When are you going to use it?' I demanded, taking a more aggressive tone.

'In the future.'

'Not good enough,' I said. And then deciding to share my thoughts. 'It's for an obituary, isn't it?'

'Well, er er–'

'It's for a fucking obituary. How could you?'

249

'I ... er ... I ... I didn't want to phone you,' she said. Her voice was quivering now, like a child terrified of being admonished. 'My producer told me to.'

'And that makes it okay, does it?' I spat. 'So let's get this right, you know Jane's got a heart condition, she's climbing a high altitude mountain: bingo! Heart attack! She dies! I know, let's get some words from Mike in advance.'

'Well, ermm ermm–'

'That's an absolute disgrace,' I said, now in full flow. 'Does the BBC not have guidelines on this? What happens when other people are in this situation? Do you ring Cherie Blair when Tony's going to Iraq – let's have an interview in the bag just in case he croaks.' I realised I was shouting, my heart was pumping and my hand was clenched in a fist.

'I'm sorry I've upset you, Mike,' the voice said quietly.

'I can't believe you called. You should have refused,' and with that I replaced the receiver. I knew I was close to tears.

'Did I hear that right. Who was it?' Darren asked.

'BBC.'

'Heartless bastards,' he said.

'Heartless bastards indeed.'

Steven had really missed his mum but was looking forward to having a conversation with her during the two-way satellite link. Sky had promised some private time after their live interview and Jane knew we'd be able to see her, but the surprise was she would also be able to see us on a monitor. When the idea had been mooted, I'd deliberated on whether Jane's mental state would be affected seeing Steven on his birthday on a monitor nearly a thousand miles away. Was the five minutes worth the mental anguish which would surely follow?

Rebecca, Steven and I lined up on the living-room sofa, a camera fixed on a tripod before us, a small six-inch monitor resting on the coffee table in front.

'When you speak to your mum, look at the camera, not the monitor,' the engineer said.

'Why?' Steven asked.

'Well, you will see your mum's mouth move before you hear the words and it'll get confusing.'

'Oh.' Steven shuffled on the couch, his eyes wide as he watched the engineer fiddle with the cable that was stretching out of the room through the front door and out to the satellite truck parked outside.

'There'll also be a delay when you speak to each other so be careful not to interrupt,' he said. It seemed a risky operation as most Tomlinson conversations were based on continual inter-ruptions. Morris, one of our two cats, strolled in stretching his back legs as if waking from an afternoon sleep.

'Becca!' Steven said, in a disapproving tone.

Rebecca cuffed Steven gently. 'What?'

'Oi, get off,' he said.

'Becca,' I said. 'Where's Morris come from? He's meant to be shut in your bedroom.'

Rebecca fixed me with a stare, and getting up

251

from the couch muttered something inaudible. Clicking her fingers, she shouted 'Food' over at Morris and he followed her obediently to the kitchen.

John, the engineer, plugged a cable into the monitor and it sprang into life showing blue sky and the Mediterranean in the background; it was a different world to the overcast afternoon in Rothwell. Seconds later Rob's voice could be heard while the camera refocused.

'Where's Mum?' Steven asked.

'She'll be here soon,' John said. Steven crouched down lower, leaning his head down as though trying to see around the corner of the monitor. Jane's voice boomed out.

'I can see her!' Steven shouted. 'I can hear her!'

'We all can, Steven,' Rebecca said dismissively. My heart went out to Steven as he sat forward on the couch, his bottom perched precariously close to the edge. Luke walked across the screen oblivious to the fact that we could see him and within seconds Jane appeared and I thought Steven was going to reach out to try to touch her.

'Mum!' Steven called, oblivious to the fact she couldn't hear him. 'Mum!' he shouted louder.

The conversation both on-air and off with Jane was difficult to say the least, the sound delay causing numerous interruptions. And while it was lovely to hear and see her, it brought it home to me that it was no substitute for touching her.

Jane dabbed at her eyes, unable to hide the tears and instinctively I knew we'd done the wrong thing by agreeing to do the interview. Jane's spirit would be crushed having seen us back home. I just hoped that the knowledge that she'd be home soon would be sufficient.

As the link finished Steven slouched back on the couch and I pulled him towards me, his head cradling against my chest. I felt his head move gently as he sobbed into my jumper.

'It's all right,' I said, gently ruffling his soft hair. 'We'll see her on Sunday.' Rebecca got up, pulling a face at Steven.

'Wuss,' she said, but I could see in her face that she was feeling exactly the same way as her little brother.

'It's okay to be sad, Steven,' I said, trying to take away any embarrassment.

'I'm not,' he growled and turned the television on.

JANE

Pulling on my still damp cycling kit, I pushed my nightclothes and toiletry bag back into the suitcase to pack into the car. The Sky crew helped us by transferring some of our luggage, the rest we carried on the bike ourselves. I was weary. We'd been cycling for eight days and had spent most of that time in rain showers.

Today, we were heading down the coastal roads. We had covered 460 miles – almost a quarter of our total distance – with an average of fifty-seven miles a day.

'Just fifty miles today,' I said to Luke as we checked our panniers and pulled on our gloves. Turning on the GPS navigation system I glanced

253

down at the map.

'It's our last whole day in Italy today, isn't it?'

I nodded at him, 'Yes, I'll be glad to eat something other than pasta and pizza.'

'I've really enjoyed it. I know it's not the case but it feels like the first half of the journey is over with.'

We quickly settled into a cycling rhythm and sailed down the coastal roads and up, keeping the sea to our left. Cars and buses passed us, leaving us in the trail of their exhaust fumes, but at least the sky was blue and our kit dried on us in the first few miles. The road was clean of debris at the edge and was smooth without ruts and potholes. The bike moved smoothly through tunnels along cliffs that fell sheer to the sea, so that we finished our day's cycling by early afternoon.

I felt more rested but still despondent as we set off for Alassio. It was Luke's birthday and the sun was glorious. There was a cool breeze from the sea as we passed through San Remo. We stopped at a café for yet another of the milky coffees that had sustained us through our Italian leg of the journey.

Sitting looking over the marina, I gave Luke his birthday gift. Some pink striped tights to go with his pink Giro T-shirt. Luke's face glowed and he pulled on the tights, and did a little dance on the pavement by the café. He sat and pulled them down. 'I know we're no substitute for your family, but we wanted to give you a small gift. We should go out and celebrate tonight,' I said.

Luke nodded. 'That would be great.'

Then it was once more on the bike, heading for the French-Italian border. We coasted through a long tunnel and then came to the border control. The buildings were empty and we stopped at the other side.

'That's one leg of the journey over,' Luke said.

'It feels really good but there's still so far to go,' I replied. We looked back along the coastline we'd just travelled and down to the road we had yet to pass.

Naturally, entering France meant we had to take on board small cultural changes. No longer were we following signs for 'Il Centro', but 'Centre Ville' and instead of stopping to drink café latte, it was café crème or café au lait. For me, the language was more familiar. I'd struggled with Italian, but Mike and I had taken some classes in conversational French so I could pick out more words when someone addressed us.

In Monaco, though, we hardly needed to speak French there were so many ex-pats. I had barely stepped out of the hotel when a grey-haired elegantly dressed woman about to cross the road spotted me. 'Jane Tomlinson?' she asked. I looked at her. 'It is, isn't it? I've been following your journey.' She put her arm round my shoulder. 'You must come and meet my sister.' And before I could protest she led me, arm still round my shoulder, across the road to a nearby pedestrian precinct where her sister was serving a customer in their craft shop.

'You know Jane,' she said to her sister, who was looking slightly perplexed at my arrival. 'We've been watching her on the television.' The sister's eyes widened as she recognised me and I shook hands with both of them. 'It's a marvellous thing you're doing,' the sister said. 'Where's your brother? We think he must be a very lovely man to support you like this.'

'Oh, Luke's headed off to the marina to look at the boats and follow some of the Grand Prix route,' I said. 'I was too tired to walk around much. I was just trying to find a postcard and then I'm off back to the hotel for a rest.' We chatted for a few more minutes and then I said, 'Well, I'll have to get back now. It was good to meet you.' I shook hands with them and left. A little spooked by the experience, I left buying the postcard till another day and returned to the hotel and stayed in my room afterwards.

Cycling along the Riviera coast was a delight. For the first time we had a full day of sunshine and we were able to explore the luxurious promontory of Cap Ferrat, admiring another marina of gleaming boats.

Luke and I were both excited as we headed off up into the hills above Nice. We were just a few days away from cycling up Mont Ventoux – the biggest challenge of the ride – but first we had to climb up from Cagnes sur Mer to Grasse, a steep journey straight out of town up the cliff-like slopes.

Above the Col de la Faye, we were just easing down the hill in the full blazing sun when we passed a group of three cyclists. I turned and looked at them as they stopped at the roadside and then reversed to shoot back down the hill towards us.

'Hi!' called one as he pulled up alongside. 'It's great to have bumped into you. We thought we'd missed you. Do you mind if we accompany you for a while.'

'Definitely not,' Luke said. 'The company would be very welcome.' It turned out that the group were ex-pat cyclists. They had been following our journey and had been keen to try to meet us out on the road to cycle alongside us.

We turned our pedals once more and our small group started the next climb. It was good to have some company. I sat and pedalled behind Luke, listening to the chatter, as we made our way slowly up the next climb. We cycled up towards a small café that was at the top. We pulled the bikes to the side of the road and sat under woven shades to enjoy a café au lait with our new friends.

On the wall was a sign. Steve, one of the three grey-haired men, explained it to us. 'You're following the Route Napoléon,' he said, tapping the rusted white painted sign. 'This is part of the route Napoleon followed from Elba back to Paris in 1815.'

'Oh right,' said Luke. 'From here we go on to Ventoux, have you been up it?'

'Oh, yes. It's a fabulous ride,' Steve said.

'What's it like?' Luke asked.

'Well, the biggest problem is not the geology. It's only a hill. The biggest problem you can have is the weather. You can be caught in snow storms in June at the top. There can be hurricanes. Or it can be forty degrees Centigrade or it can be fifteen degrees Centigrade and raining. Plus, the weather changes dramatically. It's a mountain known for its violent temper.'

'Well, we'll have to hope that it's calm when we're on our way up.'

'Oh, I'm sure the gods will be shining on you,' Steve said.

The gods weren't shining at the Point de l'Artuby. We had started early just to see the sun rise over the Grand Canyon du Verdon but the stunning views I'd remembered from the family holiday in France were shrouded by a thick, grey mist that had risen from the damp ground. Instead of the deep tree-lined ravine we could only just make out the sides of the bridge.

'You said it was spectacular,' Luke said.

'It would be if we could see it.'

We stood looking out over the arch of the bridge that crossed the gorge and the sea of mist that lapped in layer upon layer, leaving the hilltops just visible. We weren't the only ones there. High above the dizzying depths of the gorge, a small group of people was gathering to take part in a bungee jump off the bridge that stood over 500 feet above the bottom of the gorge.

'Bonjour,' I said to the man who had wandered over the better to see our bike.

'C'est magnifique,' he said pointing at the bike.

'Oui,' I said, grinning.

'You are English?' he asked.

'Oui.'

'How far have you cycled?'

'Un mille cinq cent kilometres,' I replied.

He whistled low through his teeth. 'I have come

from Marseilles to bungee today.'

'Wow. I wish we could stay to watch,' I replied. 'Have you ever jumped before?'

'No. Never.'

'Well, bonne chance, I think.'

The sun had started to move higher in the sky and the mist slowly to dissipate, burning off as the day warmed up. Cycling along the ravine we passed other cyclists who called out their sing song 'Bonjour' – very different from the crisp 'Ciao' of Italy. The striated rock face was so tall it was dizzying to look at. We pulled up at the roadside and sat precariously on rocks just feet away from a precipitous drop. I peered over, gripping the edge of the boulder tightly, to look down at the blue ribbon of the water below.

We had just one more day's cycling before we came to the eve of the pinnacle of our journey – our ascent of Mont Ventoux. We could see the jerseys of two cyclists ahead and I could feel the cadence had increased as Luke pushed us harder and found a higher gear. The distance between us dropped till we caught up with the yellow-and-red-jacketed cyclists.

'Bonjour' we called in unison as we sailed past them and started to slow a little. I could hear the gears as the cyclists struggled to change up to chase us.

'It's Jane and Luke, isn't it?'

'Yes,' I said, surprised to hear an English – even a Yorkshire – accent.

'I'm Nick,' said one. 'That's Pete.' He pointed

behind him. 'We're from Leeds as well.'

'Everyone we meet is always from Yorkshire,' I said. Luke nodded his head in agreement.

The next few miles passed quickly as we made our way towards Sault. We cycled along an avenue of trees but the day was warm as we past through the small centre of Céreste so we pulled over to sit outside the Café de France. We sat on plastic green chairs under the shade of the veranda and enjoyed the café au lait.

'We just arrived last night,' Pete said. 'We were hoping to climb Mont Ventoux tomorrow.'

'So are we,' Luke said. 'It's the highlight of the trip for me.'

'Well, we were looking up on the website yesterday before we set off and it said Mont Ventoux was shut.'

'What?' Luke exclaimed.

'No way. Are you sure?' I asked.

'It said there was too much snow on the top.'

'When we flew out we could see the snow on the Alps and I remember laughing about it.'

Luke looked stunned. I was shocked. It hadn't occurred to us that Ventoux might be closed, and we hadn't made any alternative plans. We discussed it for a while and on balance decided that we'd take our chance and carry on our way over the high plains towards the foothills of Ventoux.

Six miles later and we had our first puncture. I sat at the side of the road and watched as Luke's deft fingers manoeuvred the tyre and tube. It was quickly repaired and we set off again.

260

Fifteen minutes later, Luke stopped pedalling. 'There it is,' he said.

I looked over from behind him and there, towering above the treetops, was a large hump of white-topped rock. It rose above the rest of the high plains, nothing else around it matched it in size.

'Oh, my God,' I said. 'It's monstrous. It overshadows everything.'

'Is that snow?' Luke said.

'No, that's just the exposed limestone.'

'I bet it feels even bigger when we're climbing up it tomorrow,' Luke said.

'It's going to be hard work if it's this warm,' I said.

Luke and I stood and stared. You could just make out the white tower of the weather station at the very summit. If we had a good morning of cycling we would be at the top before midday.

MIKE

'We're going to Fraaance. We're going to Fraaance!' Steven was on the phone, chanting to Suzanne. 'We're going to Fraaance. We're going to Fraaance!'

'Pass me the phone, Steven,' I said.

I put the phone to my ear, 'We're going to Fraaance! We're going to Fraaance!' I chanted.

'Shut up, fat man,' said Suzanne. It was nine thirty on a Sunday morning and we figured she'd have the obligatory student hangover. 'Will you text me when you get there?'

261

'No probs. We're going to Fra–' Her patience exhausted, she had hung up. Although we'd offered to take her with us, she intimated that pressure of coursework meant she'd have to stay in Hull. I don't think even she believed that. The reality was that term finished in a few days and she was frightened of missing the end-of-term celebrations.

Stepping out of the plane at Nice was like walking into a sauna. There was a clear aqua-blue sky and the sun's rays reflected off the concrete causing a heat haze two foot off the ground. The French customs were extremely inefficient and it took over an hour for the passengers of one small plane to exit via the passport control.

'Dad.' Steven shook my arm, but I ignored him as I scoured the arrival hall looking for the car rental desk.

'Dad!' he said again.

'What are you looking for?' Rebecca asked.

'The Hertz desk,' I said.

'It's there!'

'Dad!' Steven tugged again.

'Yes.' I looked down at him.

'Look! Does that sign say Michael Schumacher?' Looking across there was a suited chauffeur holding out an A4 card with a name across it.

'It'll be someone else with that name, Steven.'

'Can we wait and see?'

'Divvy,' said Rebecca and we set off, forgetting it was the Monaco Grand Prix in seven days.

After a couple of hours' drive we arrived in Sault. We searched the town for the hotel, carefully manoeuvring the car to avoid the steady stream of cyclists returning from the climb to Ventoux.

Reaching a cobbled square, Steven shouted, 'There!' and I looked at him to see he was pointing to a van with a satellite dish. On top, a cable stretched from the van to across the road to where Jane was perched on a wall. It was the first time I'd seen her in seventeen days and she seemed to have physically shrunk. The cycling gear which had been so snug only two weeks before was now flapping loosely round her thighs and upper arms. She had a comedy cycling tan: ten very noticeably white fingers at the end of tanned forearms.

Parking the car, we got out and walked to a café table within yards of where Jane was concentrating on her interview. As the afternoon sun warmed my face, I realised that none of Steven's normal clothes were suitable for the 80 degree heat in the South of France. I'd packed for December in Newcastle.

Luke was seated at a table festooned with espresso cups, cycling helmets and gloves. He spotted us and waved us over, shouting, 'Hi, you lot.' Jane was still seated on the low wall chatting to the camera with ease. The land behind her fell away leading to a long valley stretching for several miles before Mont Ventoux filled up the backdrop; its huge physical presence completely dominating the landscape. My eyes were drawn to its slopes. The top looked as though it was covered in snow and ice.

Jane eventually saw us and purposefully

marched over, hugging Steven and Rebecca and asking them whether they wanted an ice cream. She looked down at them both as if seeing them for the first time, then walked to me and embraced me, her sweat-covered arms glistening in the sun. It felt as if she had come alive again after the months of chemo.

At the hotel the proprietor had reluctantly agreed to serve food despite his initial protestation that 'Zi hotel has no food on Sundays.' After various shrugs and tuts, plates of bread appeared. People (sixteen) outnumbered pieces of bread (fourteen), so within virtually a nanosecond the plates had emptied. They were replaced three times over with an ever-increasing look of disgust. There was no need to consult a menu as the choice was Hobson's and by eight thirty the kitchen was closed and the bar never opened.

As I watched Jane fuss over her nightly routine, I noticed that her appearance had changed considerably in seventeen days. Comedy tan aside, her hair was growing back quickly, bouncing into life like a spring uncoiled for the first time in months. She fussed over Steven, eyeing him up and down like a buyer snagging a new house.

'He's fine,' I told her.

'He's grown.'

'In two weeks, I doubt it.' Rebecca came in, her eyes bloodshot, the skin surrounding them puffed up like a boxer at the end of a title fight: hayfever.

'How's the revision, Becca?' Jane asked.

'Okay, I suppose.'

'When's your first exam?'

'Thursday.'

Jane looked at me as Rebecca settled next to her textbooks. 'And Dad's cooking?'

'Good,' Rebecca said.

'Steven?'

'It is, Mum, honest,' he said without his eyes deviating from the Yu-Gi-Oh cards laid out in front of him on his bed. Jane looked quizzically at me, as though suspecting some mind-altering medication or bribery had been administered to the children.

'It's okay, Jane, we *can* manage without you.' I immediately regretted that. Jane's face was impassive as she moved up from our bed and went on to the balcony. I went out to join her, placing my arms gently around the top of her shoulders. Jane shrugged me away.

'Fuck off, Mike,' she muttered.

'I can cook, wash and keep the house tidy. The kids miss you. You are their mum and I could never replace you.'

'You don't know what it's like,' she said. 'I've lost my career, my future and now my family role. What is there left? I'm worthless.' She leant over the metal railing, staring out into the twilight that hid tomorrow's journey.

'We all need you, at some level,' I said. 'The house is ticking over, we're surviving but it's not the same.' I moved closer.

'Don't complain. It's no picnic here.'

'I'm not complaining. Just explaining. But whatever I say won't be right.' I coughed again.

'Have you been to the doctor about that cough?' Jane asked.

'No, Mum.' Jane frowned and we held each other. 'I'm sorry, you must be dead tired. It's just so wonderful to see you. I love you.'

'It's very stressful here and I feel quite alone; I'm so glad to see you all.' Both of us realised how ridiculous the exchange was but more importantly even at this time of night Jane had work to do.

I woke to the sound of a rodent scrabbling on the floor. It was a relief to find it was only Jane repacking her panniers. Sunlight was streaming through the open window where all last night's washing had been removed.

'Hi,' I said.

'Morning! You slept well.' I looked up and saw Steven looking across, his head resting on the pillow.

'Are you going to breakfast?' I asked Jane.

'We've eaten. I'm just going to do a "live".'

'Oh,' I said. Jane stood up, already dressed in her cycling attire which had become like a uniform, short-sleeved T-shirt highlighting how defined her arm muscles had become. 'Where's Becca?'

'Getting a shower.'

'Has she eaten as well?'

'No,' Jane grabbed her bum bag and strapped it around her waist. 'I thought you'd appreciate a lie-in.'

'Come on, Steven, let's get moving,' I said. 'We'll grab some breakfast while you do your media, Jane.' A scowl at me and she was gone. I scurried around eating breakfast, packing, checking out, loading the hire car to ensure we were at the roadside for the day's departure. Jane and Luke set off with a real aggression. It was as though they were throwing down the gauntlet to the mountain, 'Call yourself a fucking hill?'

There was absolutely no vulnerability or suggestion of failure about Jane as the two of them picked up momentum as the road swept downhill and out of town. Once gone, Steven, Rebecca and I returned to the hotel to enjoy a coffee in the beautiful courtyard shrouded from the early morning heat.

After forty-five minutes we began following in Jane's tracks on the road to Ventoux. Twelve miles later and there was still no trace of them. The road already had started to climb so sharply that we were in first gear as we accelerated out of every hairpin bend. There were five cyclists riding with Jane today: Martyn, Maggie and Bruce from the *Yorkshire Post* and a father and son from Huddersfield who'd recognised Jane from the day before and asked to go along. It was with some relief when eventually Maggie came into view.

'Dad, where's Mum?' Steven asked looking perturbed.

'Dunno. Ahead,' I said and just then I noticed the Yorkshire Television crew running to their car some fifty yards in front. I pulled up alongside. 'Have you seen Jane?'

Phil Iveson shouted from the driving seat, 'Just ahead there – not half tonking on.'

'Cheers, Phil,' I called and I accelerated away. Two hairpins later, the tandem appeared and I hit the horn. Luke put his thumb up and Jane's head turned, no smile just sheer concentration,

267

her legs pumping up and down, every muscle as taut as a snare drum. They were eating the road, closing down on a couple of recreational riders ahead who were wearing the uniform of the US Postal Service.

I stopped a hundred yards ahead but barely had time to put the handbrake on before they were past – their rhythmic turning of the pedals like the pistons of a steam engine, pumping in unison. At Sault the previous evening, the guidebook to Ventoux suggested the ride couldn't be achieved on a tandem. Jane's response: 'I'd like to beat two hours,' she said. 'That's the average time.'

As we leapfrogged Jane for a second time, we caught and passed Martyn and Bruce. We'd passed the snow barrier some time ago and it was clear we were about to head out of the shaded area of the climb.

Bruce pulled over. 'Hi, Mike, where's Lia?'

'She was having a coffee in Sault. She was going to give Jane an hour's head-start.' Bruce looked anxious. 'What's wrong?'

'Can you ring her? She's got my camera. If Jane continues at this pace she'll get to the summit before Lia gets here.'

'I've already tried but there's no reception on the hill.'

'Oh.' Clearly irritated, Bruce rode off.

'Don't worry, Bruce. It'll be last minute but she'll get here – she always does.'

As Jane arrived, Steven, Rebecca and I sprinted alongside the tandem waving and shouting, 'Allez, allez' but after twenty yards we were already dropping behind. I'd never been prouder of Jane as I watched her and Luke plough up the road. This wasn't a middle-aged cancer patient cycling up this mountain, but a perfect, super-fit cyclist whose bike was just an extra extension of her body.

JANE

'So what do you think?' Martyn said, pointing towards Ventoux behind us.

'I'm really nervous,' I said, 'but ready to try to get up it in one go.'

'Why are you doing this anyway?' asked Ian, the reporter.

I shrugged. 'It seemed obvious. Cycling through Italy and then France, we had to climb this hump of hills. This is such a fantastic climb, I've read about it in so many books, that it was too good an opportunity to miss.'

My back had been bothering me for most of the trip. The deep-seated pain at the very lowest part of my back ached and ached. I had lost sensation down my left upper thigh, but I had managed to cycle all this way, and I wasn't going to let my aching body stop me from making this climb to the top of the mountain.

At 9 a.m. we rolled out of the town of Sault and passed a blue-edged sign on the road for the Col du Mont Ventoux. The green sign 'Ouvert' confirmed what we had been told the day before at the hotel, that the road was open, allaying our fears that we would have to find another route to ride.

After a small downhill section the climbing started. The cap of Mont Ventoux had been clearly visible all morning, a stark point on the horizon. Now we were in the foothills, the peak had disappeared. It was there lurking unseen behind the green trees that shaded the lower part of our climb.

The ride was twenty-six kilometres, about fifteen miles, and by the roadside stood yellow and white kilometre markers showing the altitude to which we had climbed. We past marker nine and Luke pointed at it.

'I can't believe we're here,' I said. 'You know when you've been talking about something for so long...'

We glided along the road, climbing steadily, our legs moving smoothly, the excitement of the day pushing us onwards and moving us swiftly up the lower reaches. The sun shone and the haze made the road in front wobble before us as we reached a small parking area with plaques by the roadside. Mike stood there, clad in a pink Giro T-shirt. Steven was alongside him with his pink Giro hat on. 'Well done. Twelve kilometres to go!' called Mike.

Luke dropped a gear and we sped along again. We were silent as we cycled. Cars passed us and then several minutes later we were overtaking Mike again, who was running alongside us as we moved past him at speed. 'Go, Jane, go,' I heard him cry from behind.

Luke and I laughed aloud, both excited, as we continued the climb. We reached Le Chalet Reynard, nestled into the hillside, a white stone building with only a few stunted shrubby trees surrounding it. That meant we only had another six kilometres more of the climb.

As we passed, I saw the cyclists Pete and Nick from the day before mount their bikes and set off on the last section up to the top. We had left the shelter of the trees and the true spirit of Ventoux was now evident. The road was just a grey stripe along the yellow-white rocky hillside that dropped steeply away to one side and climbed dizzyingly on the other. We sped up the first bend and then moved more slowly as the gradient became gradually steeper till we had dropped to the smallest climbing ring on the tandem and our pedalling rate dropped. The bike grew heavier and heavier as the climb tested us to our limits. We passed red-and-white-striped snow gates, plough markers black and yellow at the roadside. It was warm now and sweat beaded on my face and ran down into my eyes.

By now, I was panting – my breath coming in short gasps. My body was shaking, my thighs were burning. The hillside was a barren moon-scape and my vision was blurred from the salty sweat that stung my eyes. Luke pushed and pushed and the bike weaved with all our efforts.

We passed the memorial for Tommy Simpson that I'd seen on our holiday. There were several people stood alongside and it was littered with colourful bike debris. Only one more kilometre to go and we would finish.

'Are we going to get up all the way?' I asked Luke, panting with effort. He nodded and our legs pushed round and round.

The road here was a dark black, the new surface smooth beneath the tyres. Beside us, the gunmetal grey of the crash barriers protected us from the sheer drop on the other side. I was struggling to breathe in, the air hot, drying my mouth. The white stones surrounding us bounced the heat back up off the mountainside making us warmer and warmer.

Down the hillside I could see dark ravines visible where water had channelled and travelled down the hill, with nothing to heed its path. The weather station was directly before us, but we still had several more snaking hairpin bends to climb before we reached the summit. The road was patchy here, faded names of other visitors scrawled beneath us as we passed slowly over their graffiti.

'Don't ... want ... to ... do this ... tomorrow ... again,' I panted.

'Once ... is enough,' Luke panted back.

Luke's back was bent low, his shoulders hunched, his body moved from side to side. I focused on the tip of his helmet and the road below the front wheel, willing us to move forward, pushing away the pain from my legs as we slowly crept up and up.

Finally, we crawled over the last hairpin. Round the bend was the very top. I could see people gathered and felt relief that we had made it. We eased slowly towards our finish point.

There we were at the summit. We lifted our hands and cheered. The Mont Ventoux climb lay behind us, before us the rest of our journey. We had taken one and half hours, much less than we had thought it would take. 'Well done, Luke,' I said. 'Thank you.' I reached forward to put my hand on his shoulder. And he nodded his acknowledgement.

I could see Nick to my left. He had already finished and had waited to see us complete our climb.

Mike ran over to us as I was climbing from the bike. 'You made it,' he said. There were tears in his eyes. Seeing him, I stepped forward and his arms enveloped me. Tears ran their silent course down my face.

'I'm still here,' I thought. 'Nine months ago I didn't know if I'd even be able to return to Mont Ventoux. Now I've cycled it. Another goal. Another dream.'

CHAPTER 8

May 2004

MIKE

After the adrenalin rush and emotion of the climb up Ventoux, I had to admit that the journey to Nyons in the valley north of the mountain was something of an anticlimax. Nestled in the bottom of a steep valley, the pretty town appeared on our left and we entered via a busy sun-drenched road. It was about 2 p.m. – the early start meant we still had most of the day to spend with Jane.

We drove into a beautiful square, more Italian in design than French, which probably harked back to a time when it was under control of a different nation. The square was open, large and empty; I peered around and was disappointed not to see our hotel.

'Are we here yet?' Steven asked. He was becoming restless. Poor lad, in the few days we'd been here he'd suffered the indignity of having his winter jumper and long trousers swapped for a pink Giro d'Italia T-shirt, a baseball cap and some cheap kids' sunglasses – the type where the arm would snap within a day.

'Yes,' I said. 'We just need to find the hotel. It's called the Hotel Valouse – will you look out for it for me?'

'Okey dokey, my man,' he said.

'Stop it, Steven,' Rebecca said. 'Your stupid talk makes you sound like a right wally.' She clicked the ring file of her folder and put down her revision notes.

'What?' Steven said with his arms outstretched Tony Blair-style as if protesting his innocence.

I surveyed the square, eyes peeled for the Hotel Valouse, but it was no use. There was no sign of it. Noting the time and the fact that Steven needed a drink, we parked up and went to the nearest *bar tabac* for a croque-monsieur and a coke. On leaving, I asked for directions to the hotel, but received an Eric Cantona shrug from the waiter. Bearing in mind that his English had been word perfect when I'd ordered the food, I smelt a French rat.

We wandered around the square, asking several

strangers, 'Ou est l'Hotel Valouse?' But they would either shrug or speak so quickly I had no chance of understanding them. After we'd thanked them, I'm sure I heard the word *Anglaise* followed by laughter and the choreographed shrug. Feeling defeated I phoned Rob from Sky to ask him for any more details of the hotel name and Street.

'It must be there, Mike,' he said.

'I can't find it.'

He sighed. 'Look, I'll be there soon myself. Is there a tourist information?' I could sense he thought me feckless, in a small town how could I not find a reasonably sized hotel?

'Closed for the afternoon.' Within thirty minutes of one o'clock the town had shut up, and the streets were deserted. 'I'll keep looking.'

I grabbed Steven's hand, leaving Rebecca on a bench in the square and I widened our search to include the surrounding streets. Eventually, we found a proprietor of a small convenience store who not only spoke English, he had a local map and was willing to help. His finger hovered over Nyons then slowly he began to trace a road eastwards several inches over the map. My eyes flicked to see the scale but couldn't locate it.

'Is it far?' I asked.

'Thirty kilometres,' he said. I gasped, thinking of Jane.

When I phoned Rob and told him, he was sceptical. 'Thirty kilometres? Is he sure?' Within minutes Rob was phoning back. 'It's bloody miles, Mike, it's not in Nyons, its Hôtel Valouse in Valouse – it's a completely separate town.'

By the time I returned to the car and found it

on the Collins road map it was clear that it was at least twenty kilometres further up the valley, with the final six leading to a cul de sac with what looked like an unforgiving steep hill.

Jane was philosophical when I called. 'These things happen,' she said. Even so, I knew that her legs that were already stiff and cramped and another twenty kilometres was only going to exacerbate the problem.

Rob and I took our cars up the main valley road heading for Serres before turning off left following the River Bentrix and finally heading left to Valouse. It looked to be a tough ride because of a number of little sharp climbs, but the hotel was in a beautiful, quiet, green valley, worlds away from the moonscape of Ventoux. There was even an outside pool – something of a luxury after the basic auberges we'd been staying in previously. With Jane planning her and Luke's 'rest day' for the whole of tomorrow, a more perfect spot she could not have chosen.

We checked in, unloaded the bags and were having a coffee relaxing under a canopy of vegetation at the front of the hotel when Jane arrived. Although tired, there was no disguising her delight at successfully climbing Ventoux as the smile never left her face. After showering and washing her kit, she joined the other thirteen of us and we went to eat in the hotel restaurant where bowl after bowl of bread was demolished.

By evening, Steven was flaked out in his bed. I tucked his skinny topless torso under a sheet and ruffled his matted hair. Rebecca was outside chatting to Lia, the conversation punctuated by various girly giggles. Jane moved carefully around the room, ducking to avoid the low ceilings, methodically sorting her cycling kit. Some of it was hanging outside on a line, some was soaking in the sink, some carefully folded on the bed.

'Has it been worth it, Mike?' she asked, as she began to wring some of the clothes in the sink.

'What?' I lay on the bed, my hands behind my head. 'The ride?'

'Is it worth it, all the effort, what's it for?'

I sensed it was a rhetorical question so I didn't say anything. My mind was distracted already thinking of the drive back to Nice tomorrow and the flight home.

'I miss you all dreadfully,' Jane said.

'I know.'

'I'm not doing this again. I don't want to be away from you all.' Her eyes moistened, the hard veneer cracked and I stood up and held her.

'You'll see Suzanne next week, me and Steven the week after.' A tear gently rolled down her cheek and I wiped it away. 'It'll be worth it, we'll raise a lot of money.'

A kind of gloom had set in over the last few days. We knew after last year's John o'Groats ride to expect it, but that made it no less easier to deal with. We had questioned at length whether it was right for Jane to be away from the family for five weeks. But there was no correct answer, no magical solution, so we were left to make the decision that was best for everyone. It was a charity bike ride and its sole purpose was to make money so that those cancer and children's charities we support could make a difference to people who were in a worse position than ourselves; the only measure of the success was how much was in the bank at the end of the ride.

'No more, Mike,' Jane whispered, her head resting softly on my chest. 'This is it. I'm finished.' I held her tight, knowing that nothing I could say would help.

JANE

We had enjoyed a celebratory meal at Valouse with Mike, Rebecca and Steven, and others who had joined us for the Ventoux ascent. The next day was a rest day and after Mike had left I was able to walk and explore our resting spot. Hameau de Valouse was a peaceful haven, an isolated group of stone farmhouses and cottages set in a small vale with a clear bubbling stream running through it. A short walk down the lane led to a small pasture full of wild flowers. I lay on my front to examine an undisturbed orchid, its purple flower low and almost hidden in the grass. The exhilaration of the climb the day before was still with me but I missed home, the normality of everyday life, cooking meals for the family, walking out to the local shops. Here, everything changed every day, nothing remained the same.

Alas, we were many miles from home and, after a day's rest, Luke and I left the tranquillity of the hamlet to head towards Chabeuil through the rolling hills and the limestone countryside of Gorges de Trente-Pas. As we cycled, we could hear the gentle bubble and fizz of the stream by the roadside and the musical clangs of the sheep bells from the hills. The wind moved bright red poppies in the fields, waving them like jewels through the golden grasses.

Arriving at Chabeuil after cycling through such beautiful scenery was a disappointment. A tired hotel next to a road that was all concrete and reflected heat. It drove us from our beds early the next morning to reach Lyons before the day became too warm. We'd been on the road for eighteen days, cycling for seventeen of them. Already the memory of our day of relaxation at Valouse seemed distant and before us there were many more days of cycling still in France.

Lyons was busy. It was the Feast of the Ascension and a public holiday in France. Luke stepped out of the hotel, while I relaxed in a shower. Pulling on dry clothes, I lay on the bed dozing, wishing I had something to feed my gnawing hunger.

The door swung open. 'Here you go. Which do you want, chicken or cheese?' Luke said, tossing a small carrier bag at me.

'Oh, chicken, please. You read my mind, I'm starving.'

'How about a bit of people-watching later? We can walk into town for a burger.'

'That would be great.'

'You look done in though. Why don't you rest for a while?'

I nodded and finished chewing at my sandwich. Laying my head back on the pillow I drifted into a place just before sleep, listening to the drone of French voices accompanying a black and white slapstick French film that Luke was laughing loudly at.

The light had dimmed outside but my head was clearer, my eyes less heavy. I swung my legs over the side of the bed.

Luke looked up. 'Ready for a walk out?' he said.

'Yes, I'm feeling much better thanks.'

'How far did we cycle today?'

I looked at my scribbled notes. 'Seventy miles with a maximum speed of forty-one and a half miles per hour. We had an average of twelve and a half miles per hour.'

'Go on, then, tell me how far it is tomorrow.'

'Do you really want to know?'

'Yes.'

'Roughly one hundred miles – a little more.'

Luke raised his eyebrows. 'Why?'

'What do you mean?'

'Why are we cycling one hundred miles tomorrow?'

I smiled at him and pulled on a yellow jacket and moved towards the door.

'Just to prove we can,' I said.

The alarm shrieked. It was 5 a.m. and I turned towards it, reached out my hand, fumbled and knocked it on to the floor. Leaning out of the bed, I cursed and reached for the clock and silenced it. I found the light switch and brightened the dark room. I pulled on my cycling shorts and tops and went into the bathroom, washing my face and brushing my teeth. I smeared on Sudocrem liberally. I knew I was lucky not to have any saddle sores yet after nineteen days on the road.

When I'd finished in the bathroom, I found Luke waiting to carry out his ablutions. I pushed my non-cycling clothes back into the suitcase and pulled on my shoes, fastening them with difficulty. The fingertips of three of my fingers on my left hand were tingling and had little other sensation, which made even the smallest task of tying my shoelaces difficult. This was due to the chemotherapy damaging the nerves, and exacerbated by the daily cycling putting pressure on the palms of my hands.

A sudden arc of light pierced the still dim room as Luke checked the bike lamps that we would need at this early hour.

'How long do you reckon it will take?' Luke asked.

'I reckon about eight hours, looking at how fast we can cycle,' I replied.

We manoeuvred the heavy touring tandem from the rear courtyard through the hotel lobby and out of the front door.

'Foot up,' he said and moments later we were cycling through the darkened streets of Lyons, heading for the centre and then the hills to the north.

'It's the next right over the river,' I called to Luke and my voice echoed in the silent city. We followed a small white truck over the River Rhône and were surprised when a man alighted from the rear of it, jumping clear and sprawling himself untidily on to the pavement.

'Bah!' he called after the truck and picked himself up, gesticulating before turning and winking at us.

We crossed the second river of Lyons – the River Saône – and moved into the old quarter of the city. The cobbled streets opened into squares as we cycled through.

'Oh, look, another hill,' Luke said flatly as we started our slow ascent out of the city.

'Stop moaning,' I panted back at him.

He didn't reply and we concentrated on moving our heavy bike onwards and upwards. Finally, we looked back over the city. Street lamps were still lit but the sky was lightening.

We hurried on down the road and by 9 a.m. we'd reached Lamure about thirty miles further on and were ready to eat breakfast. We sat by the roadside Café de la Maine and ordered café au lait. I picked a pastry from the display but Luke had headed for the *boulangerie* at the corner. He returned with an intriguing round bun, crusted with pink jewels of almond paste and sugar.

'Were there any more?' I asked, and his eyes widened as a grin spread across his face.

'There's a huge one,' he said, opening his hands to show a large loaf size. 'Shall we get it?'

He didn't need much encouragement from me and headed back to the *boulangerie*, returning with a large round paper-wrapped bun.

'This is what I'll look like when I've eaten this,' he said and pushed the loaf under this cycling top to make a large pregnant bulge complete with lumps and bumps. He brought it back out and pulled the paper from it. He unfastened his pannier and put it on the top, pushing and pulling at other items to make it fit. Martyn, who had been watching us, walked over, peering into the pannier.

'What else is in there?' he said.

'Hey, keep your nose out, that's our food,' Luke said.

'If that's your food, what's that?' He pointed to the bag bungeed on to the pannier rack.

Luke waved the enquiring hands away. 'Oh, that's our fresh fruit.'

Martyn's eyes widened 'But–'

'But nothing ... keep your hands off, it's mine,' Luke said.

After breakfast, we cruised past a market stall of fresh flowers as we left the town. It was a journey full of magical sights. On the outskirts a red-bricked castle stood floating adrift in its moat, set back from the road, moss creeping up its water-salted walls. Castellated prominences hung over courtyards. A courtly building, grand and pro-vincial with its dome and weather vane. Small sash windows from an earlier time overlooked the byway.

Looking up the road we could see flashes ahead of us and then we heard a large crack of thunder. The road out of the village was uphill once more and seemed to go on for ever and ever as we pushed and pushed, the skies darkening with each circle of our legs until dark spots of rain started to fall.

'Flat day, flat day, me arse,' Luke remarked as we passed over the Charmieux at over 2000 feet. 'How are you feeling?'

'Fine. Really well.'

'You look like you're enjoying yourself.'

'I am. I really am. What about you?'

'Well, I'll be glad when we get there today.'

On and on, through the rain showers and sun-shine, the road spun into the distance and we raced down the black crusted highway round every bend, each hill rising harshly after our sweet singing downhill.

At last, the milometer read 100 and we'd nearly made it to Bourbon-Lancy in mid-France. Two days' cycling in one would give us the day off tomorrow – a day of not having to go anywhere near the bike.

'Yvette?' A man's melodic French voice called out from behind me. 'Ou est Yvette?'

I leant forward in my bench seat, under the arched terrace of the Grand Hôtel du Parc Thermial to see a tall man, his well-clipped beard peppered with grey, catch the hand of a young French woman. Her ivory dress was everything you would imagine of a chic French wedding – beautifully cut it showed off her tiny waist, curved hips and slim calves. Her dainty feet were clad in satin shoes. I watched as the couple made their way into the hotel, past the tall urns of drooping palm trees.

The pump from the thermal baths squeaked at regular intervals as I resumed my reading, en-joying my full day without cycling. I glanced at my watch and closed my book, picking up my bag containing my swimming costume. I had some treatments booked at the Thermes de Bourbon-Lancy – 'source eternelle de bien être'.

The reception area was light and airy and

modern, there was soothing music playing over speakers, and the white-clad receptionist smiled at me as I stepped forward with the card that showed the treatments I had booked.

In the treatment room, lying on my front, hot, smooth stones were placed on my legs and I was left alone. I felt myself relax to the calming soothing music and drifted into my own thoughts.

My whole body felt rejuvenated as I stepped out of the thermal baths and made my way back to the hotel.

'Don't you know what a rest day means?' I asked Luke. He was cycling round the courtyard of the hotel, checking out the bike someone had loaned him for the day.

'I'm off into the hills for an hour,' he said. 'This bike feels so light after the tandem. What are you going to do?'

'I thought I'd go and have a look at the old town and have some lunch, then rest.'

'That sounds like a plan. I'll catch up with you later.' He turned the pedals and made his way out of the tall gates.

I set off up the steep hill. Tall beamed town-houses either side of the cobbled lane crowded into each other. The sign above the antique shop creaked and squeaked with the wind.

I paused at a dark oak-coloured restaurant, Le Grignott, its small window revealing tables set with fine white cloths. I looked down the menu and pushed the door open. It was a simple lunch of omelette and salad followed by 'crêpe avec jus du citron' and washed down with 'café crème grand'. I ate in silence and watched a young French family enjoying their meal. The toddler sat in a high chair solemnly eating his lunch and only crying when his mother moved his plate before he'd finished every last morsel.

Full and relaxed, I headed back down the lane to the hotel.

The next day, rejoining the road heading northwards from Bourbon-Lancy, the hills rolled on and up and then swooped down. Large trucks rocked the bike as they pulled by us and we soon left for quieter lanes running by rivers and the canal networks. Cows and calves turned heavy-lashed eyes towards us as we cycled slowly by. A glance to reassure themselves and then they turned back to their pasture.

Black lanes turned to red-tarmacked roads, heavy under the tyres of the bike, the borders softened by the long waving grasses bending down. We passed by the arched bridge, over the Canal du Nivernais. The ancient plaque said it was built in 1837. We sat in front of the Château de Châtillon en Bazois, a tall house with long slender chimneys reaching up to the skies. As we ate our lunch of boiled eggs and bread purloined from the breakfast table at the hotel, we admired the long terraced garden reaching down to the canal.

Over the next day, we followed the canal paths northwards through France, which were rutted but free of traffic, quiet and calm.

'Have you seen that heron?' I asked Luke. He turned and looked as the tall bird pushed itself upwards and followed us further down the waterway. 'It's been trailing us for ten minutes or more.'

'It must be wondering what we are. If it's got a nest round here it'll want to make sure we don't go near it,' Luke said. Our heron soon lost interest as we moved further on.

'What's that sound?' I asked Luke. I could hear a continuous little sshhhh every time the wheel revolved.

Luke shook his head. 'I can't hear anything.'

We continued on. 'No, it's definitely not right, it sounds like something rubbing,' I said.

'I'll check it out next time we stop,' Luke said. We stopped sooner than anticipated, Luke suddenly braking and pulling into the side of the road. He leapt of the bike and snatched at his helmet and glasses.

'Has it gone?' he asked, as a large fly, momentarily dazed by its collision with Luke's face, recovered and sped off with a noisy buzz of wings.

'Yes,' I said, trying not to laugh. Luke pawed at his face.

'That was a bit of a girly thing to do,' he admitted.

'You should have seen yourself,' I said and couldn't contain myself any longer and bent over with laughter.

'Yeah, yeah,' he said, 'let's check this bike out.' We removed the panniers and upended the bike. 'Yes, I can see the problem. We'll need to replace this tyre.' The tyre wall had collapsed a little and bulged alarmingly at the side. The bike was heavy; the rear of the bike with the panniers put a lot of weight through that tyre.

Our overnight stop was at Clamecy, a picturesque town in mid-France. I was beginning to be in awe of all the beautiful towns we had visited, it was no wonder the locals seemed so proud.

As Luke repaired the bike that evening, I walked towards a weir where the river cascaded noisily. The early evening sun spun the water copper colours. I walked to the side of the weir where there was an old photograph printed on to metal on the wall. It showed the river full of logs flowing down stream. Men stood astride some large ones to free the log jams and help the timbers on their way. Clamecy was clearly an old logging town.

Back on the bike we cycled in full sunshine. We were enjoying the cycling but the tedium of climbing on the bike day after day was tiring us. Then some small sight, some scenery, reminded me of how lucky I was to be there. Passing over the arched bridge of Montbuoy, I looked down to see the still water full of lilies, large white flowers cradling the yellow stamens. There was the click of the boules as we passed the elders of the town throwing the silver ball underarm with a slight flick of the wrist. The victorious cries followed us as we moved on.

At Puisaye, after a couple of hours' cycling, we stopped for coffee, sitting overlooking the main street, the warm milky coffee too good to rush.

'I think I've had enough of this cycling lark,'

Luke said.

'I know. I'm feeling worn out and really tired. I think my body is trying to tell me to get off the bike and stop,' I said.

'Another coffee?' Luke said and he headed for the dark interior of the small café.

We lingered over our second cup of coffee but could put off the moment when we had to sit ourselves back on the bike no longer. We set off through the town past the bustle of the busy market day.

'Can you hear that?' Luke asked as we cycled along another quiet lane. I could hear the trill of the birds, the rush of the wind through the trees.

'What?' I asked.

'There are no cicadas.'

I lifted my helmet strap and listened. Sure enough, the shrill chirrup of the cicadas was no longer with us. For over twenty days we had been accompanied by the monotony of the creaking calling and now, suddenly, it was as if somebody had found the off switch.

Through market towns we passed beds of watercress, some being picked and bunched for market. The orange dry soil was green with herbs. I could see marjoram and peppermint crops stretching far into the distance. The uniformity of the fields was disturbed by dark rounded boulders rolled there by glaciers many ages before.

Our stop for the night was to be Paris and, following the Canal du Loing towards the French capital, we could feel the urgency of the metropolis in the distance. The roads were busier, quicker as we followed the overhead power lines on their march to the city – great metal limbs outstretched by the roadside, the cables buzzing with the energy they carried.

The ride was relentlessly hot and the nearer we drew to Paris the more houses there were, the wider the road, and the greater the reflected heat. We pulled up outside a small *tabac* and guzzled cold cokes, the chilling liquid sweet in our dry mouths.

We came upon the Seine and followed its course, weaving our way among people strolling its banks. Hot and tired we carried on into the city. The thrill of reaching Paris was tarnished with the reality of cycling through the outskirts of the town, and then the busy streets of the city itself.

The arches alongside the riverbank offered brief respite from the sun, but soon we could cycle no further. The pavement was too narrow to take the tandem any longer.

'If we take the panniers off, we can carry it up the stairs,' Luke said, defeated.

I nodded, my chin dropping low as we heaved the bike up on to the roadside to meet the mad Parisian motorists. We crossed seven bridges before the Pont de la Concorde and then we hurried to the Place de la Concorde. We were just a short distance from our destination – the British Embassy in Paris. We had received an invitation to stop at the embassy, and suitably impressed we had accepted it.

As we passed the obelisk, Luke stared at the golden and black fountains and then pulled his attention back to the road and weaved his way through the cars.

'Left here,' I called. We were now on rue du Faubourg Saint Honoré – each foreign ambassador's residence hidden by high heavy black gates. The pavement was obstructed by cones and the whole road heavily policed.

We stopped the bike, and climbed off it opposite the British Embassy. Luke stood holding the bike as I walked towards the gates. A gendarme stepped forward and shook his head, indicating with his hand to move back.

I went back to Luke and was sitting tired on the kerbside wondering what to do when the gates swung open and we were hailed across the street by a dark-suited gentleman. The gendarme watched, his eyebrows raised, as we wheeled our dark steed through the fortified gates, heavily weighed down with our panniers, a baguette held in place with the bungee strings, evidence of our travels.

We rolled the bike up the paved entrance to the grand porticos and arched front door. A young man, black-suited with a crisp white shirt, aided us. Our helmets were strung on the handlebars, swinging as the bike moved. From the grand entrance to the building stepped a silver-haired man, who greeted us.

'I'm John Holmes, the ambassador, and this is my wife Penny.' An elegant woman, immaculately dressed, in stark contrast to myself in my cycling shorts and top, stepped forward and we shook hands.

'Nice to meet you,' I said as two dogs gambolled at our feet.

'They're very playful,' said Luke.

'Yes, meet Polly and Whiskey,' Sir John said.

'Oh they'll enjoy me. I smell revolting,' I said, only too conscious next to the smartly dressed couple of my wet clothes clinging to me and the salt marks on my cheeks and bare arms.

'How was the cycling today?' Sir John asked.

'It was a long hard slog,' I said. 'Over seventy miles into a headwind.'

'Oh, goodness me – seventy miles! You must need a rest,' said Sir John. 'Ben, our butler, will show you to your rooms.'

Ben, a young man in crisp white shirt and dark trousers, took my pannier from me. 'This is Howard, our footman,' said Ben, and Howard stepped forward and greeted us.

They led us into a magnificent reception area, its chequered marbled floor leading to a grand curved staircase. Further in, we stopped at the door of a small lift and Ben gestured with his hand. 'If you get in, we'll see you up there,' he said smiling as we stepped inside. He pressed a button and the doors slid shut hiding Ben and Howard from view.

'What is this place like?' I said to Luke, my mouth open slightly with surprise at finding ourselves in such formal and beautiful lodgings for the night. The lift ascended slowly and, when the doors opened, Ben and Howard stood before us, cool as cucumbers and not a bit out of breath despite having run up goodness knows how many flights of stairs. We were shown down a carpeted hallway to a suite of rooms.

'I'm sorry, Luke,' said Ben. 'Your room doesn't

have its own bathroom, but there's one through here.' He pointed to a separate door that lead off from the small hallway.

I was shown into my room. A huge soft bed covered with pillows dominated it. There was also a chaise longue and a large desk supplied with stationery. The bathroom was bigger than in any hotel I had stopped in. Ben and Howard then left us in our luxurious rooms.

'I feel a little underdressed,' Luke said, grinning.

'Wow,' I said as I looked around at the original paintings on the walls.

'Your own bathroom,' Luke teased. 'I'll just make do with this one then.' He opened the door on to a room that held a large bath, with plenty of soft towels on the racks.

My phone rang. 'Hi, Mum.' It was Suzanne. 'We've just arrived at our hotel. The train journey to Paris was a bit long, but we've got a fantastic room.'

'You should see mine,' I said. 'When do you want to meet?'

'Tom and I will just have a bit of a wander and then we can meet up early evening.'

'I'm looking forward to seeing you,' I said.

After showering and resting, Luke and I stepped outside the embassy and there waiting opposite the gates for me was Suzanne. Dressed in a white skirt and dark top with her makeup elegantly applied and her hair smoothed back and glossy, she couldn't have contrasted any more than with myself. My hair was growing back rapidly now from the chemo, and stuck out from my head in kinks.

'You look so grown-up,' I said and we hugged each other. Tom, her boyfriend, was standing next to her. 'Hi, Tom,' I said. 'It's great to see you both.'

We stopped in an Italian restaurant and ate large dishes of pasta washed down with a cold beer. 'So, you're coming to the embassy for dinner tomorrow?' I asked.

'You bet. Will you be able to show us your room?' Suzanne asked.

I smiled. 'For you, anything.'

By 9 p.m. I was tired. Suzanne and Tom walked back through town to show us their hotel. We left them to catch the Métro to see Montmartre, while Luke and I made our way back to the embassy. In my room, I changed straight into clean pyjamas, got into bed, and pulling back the heavy covers sunk into oblivion.

I slept soundly, but after so many days of early starts I woke early. Luke knocked on the door. 'We ought to get downstairs for breakfast,' he said.

'I'm nearly ready,' I called from the bathroom finishing rubbing myself dry and pulling on some clean clothes.

We walked down together and sat at a large circular table with other guests of the embassy. Lady Penny introduced the others and we all said hello. I forgot their names instantly, and spent the rest of the breakfast trying to disguise the fact. As I sipped at my second coffee Lady Penny turned to me.

'What were you thinking of doing today?' she asked.

'I thought I'd go to the Louvre and look around,' I said.

Luke was taking a swig of orange juice. 'I was going to take in some of the sights too,' he said. We had spent so much time in each other's company that we had agreed to do our own thing for the morning.

'If you want to look round the galleries, I'd recommend the Musée d'Orsay. It's not so vast as the Louvre, which makes it easier to look round on a short visit.'

From the embassy, it didn't take long to walk to the museum. It was a magnificent building, transformed from a railway station and opened in 1986 as a gallery. Inside, I was surprised to see how light and modern it was. Walking from room to room, I enjoyed seeing paintings that I had only experienced in books before. I stood back to look at Renoir's 'Dancing at the Moulin de la Galette', admiring the detail. Further on the brasher colours of Gauguin and Van Gogh stood out against the more natural shades of Monet's waterlilies.

Outside, the weather was kinder and the sun shone down. People sat and enjoyed sandwiches on the benches which lined the footpaths, others lay on the grass reading. I came to a small table, shaded by lime trees, and sat to eat a sandwich and watch people rushing through the gardens – maybe to meet their lovers for a few snatched moments while they lunched.

Sir John had arranged a small gathering of friends and other guests at the embassy later that day to celebrate Luke and me arriving in the capital. Sir John had asked us if we would mind cycling into the courtyard to greet the guests and so it was that Luke and I found ourselves outside the gates we'd arrived at yesterday, waiting for our cue.

Vicki, Sir John's assistant, ran down the drive. 'Can you give us five minutes?' she asked, a little breathless.

'Yes, most certainly,' Luke said and to pass the time, we turned the bike and set off to cycle round the corner and back. A few corners later Luke turned his head round to me.

'Do you know where we are?' he said.

'I'm not sure,' I said. 'I'm a bit disorientated. Try the next right and then a left.'

We sped along the narrow Paris streets becoming more and more lost. My telephone rang. 'Where are you?' Vicki asked, clearly confused.

'Ermm, good question,' I said, scanning the buildings around me for anything that looked familiar. 'We're not sure ... but we won't be long.'

We stopped pedalling and I climbed from the bike while Luke turned it round, nearly doubled with laughter.

'I don't believe we've got so lost,' I said through giggles.

'You're keeping the ambassador waiting,' Luke said, his solemn face suddenly cracking as he, too, lost himself in a fit of giggles. 'Here pass the map.'

Another couple of turns and thankfully we were back on familiar ground and soon arrived back at the entrance to the embassy. The large dark gates swung open and a small crowd of about fifty people was revealed. We came to a stop in the courtyard and Sir John stepped forward.

Our tandem was carried with great aplomb by Ben and Howard into the Embassy to reside as a guest of honour in the gallery overlooking the garden, its tyres resting on the polished marble floor. 'An enormous welcome to Jane and Luke,' said Sir John. 'They've done well to get this far and still have a long way to go. They're looking fit and well. It's great to see you.' I nodded, acknowledging his kind words. He continued, 'All the best – and I need to hand over this cheque for your charities. The monies have come from a twenty-four-hour snooker match, a fun run and many other personal donations.'

He handed over a cheque and I smiled and looked at the assembled party. 'Thank you very much,' I said. 'Thanks to you all for coming to greet us today. I feel a little underdressed.'

Luke nodded in agreement as we stood clad in cycling gear amongst the elegantly dressed crowd. 'This has been one of our highlights,' Luke said. 'You've made us very welcome.'

When the guests had left, we had an hour to dress ourselves for an evening meal with Sir John and Lady Holmes and their guests. Suzanne and Tom had stayed after the reception and sat in my bedroom looking around enviously.

I pulled my cardigan over the only dress I had

with me. We stepped downstairs for pre-dinner drinks in the red room, which was full of comfortable and elegant chairs. The room gradually filled with the other guests till there were a dozen of us chatting.

Dinner itself was nerve-racking. As guests of honour, Luke – wearing a shirt and pair of trousers brought from England by Suzanne for the occasion – and I were served first and we were all fingers and thumbs. Not wanting to make fools of ourselves, we managed through the meal by watching others, and with the whispered advice from Ben. Then we were presented with a triumph of summer puddings with pastry tandems made for us by their chef. Returning to the red room we sat and chatted with the other guests over port and coffees.

The next day the ambassador and his wife stood at the entrance to their residence. 'Good luck for the rest of your trip,' said Sir John.

'Thank you,' I said, shaking his hand and making my way to the bike, where Luke was already seated in the front saddle. 'And thank you so much for the hospitality. You've made us feel very welcome. It's a shame to be leaving.'

Luke and I were on our way once more. We glided slowly out of the driveway and back on to the street, the peacefulness of the embassy grounds shattered by the busy Parisian noise outside. Looking back at our hosts, they waved at us as we left their boundary and headed for the Place de la Concorde.

It was only minutes later that we reached the

famous bustling roundabout, a veritable circus of cars, buses and lorries all vying for space on the road. Horns beeped, engines revved. Luke brought the bike to a halt.

'Shall we go for it?' he said, grinning.

I looked straight ahead, wondering how on earth we'd make it alive. 'Yeah,' I said. 'Why not?'

We began pedalling down the long wide avenue of the Champs Elysées with four lanes of traffic spluttering alongside us. Luke was laughing as we approached the Arc de Triomphe.

'What sort of madness is that?' he said as cars streamed past us to make their way around the arch. There seemed to be no logic to the system. We knew that the cars coming on to the roundabout had right of way but it didn't stop other vehicles pulling out in front of us and beeping their horns. I looked behind to make sure no one was going to shunt us as Luke continued to navigate his way warily through the cars.

'Where are we headed?' I yelled.

'The Eiffel Tower, I think,' Luke shouted. I could barely hear him above the noise of the traffic. There were twelve exits in all and we needed to make our way almost completely round to the avenue d'Iena which ended at the Jardins du Trocadero overlooking the tower. It was an adrenalin-pumping experience but one we managed to escape unscathed.

Nothing prepares you for the vastness of the Eiffel Tower. The metal structure soaring above the river crowns the Seine.

Suzanne and Tom had made their own way to the Jardins du Trocadero to bid farewell to us.

'Safe cycling,' said Suzanne. 'See you at home, Mum.'

We hugged. I was saddened to be leaving her. I had enjoyed spending time with her, time that felt like I was sharing the company of another adult and equal.

'Uugh, you're all sweaty,' she said, pulling away and wiping her hands.

'Thanks, I know that.'

'Look after Mum,' Suzanne said to Luke.

'But of course, that's what I'm here for,' he replied.

We had sixty-five miles to cycle to our next stop, and negotiating the heavy Parisian traffic would add hours on to the journey. It was time to leave.

MIKE

Steven was sitting in his car seat stretching his neck upwards to see over the passenger seat in front of him and out of the windscreen. I had my mobile phone to my ear and had my other hand on the steering wheel as I tried to tug at my damp T-shirt which was clinging to my back with sweat. My brow was soaking wet and I frowned, concentrating. The Amiens traffic appeared to be coming at me from every angle – as though I were trapped inside some crazed computer game.

'Where are you?' shouted Jane down the phone over the loud street noise. I couldn't answer so hung up and moved the mobile away from my ear to free up my hand to drive.

'Are we there yet, Dad?' Steven asked.

I didn't respond.

'Daaad.'

'I'm just trying to find the hotel, Steven,' I said. The phone rang but I picked it up and pressed the red button again, refusing to accept the call. Within seconds it went again.

'Mike,' Jane sounded more anxious this time. 'Mike, just find the station and turn left; we're on that road.'

'Yes,' I snapped. 'I'll sort it.' I hung up again. Feeling faint and clammy, I got out of the car, coughed violently and leant against the car roof. I had still not been able to shift the fever I'd been suffering from for the last six weeks.

I got back inside and after a couple of minutes we were in the busy square of Amiens station where we turned left and in the distance was a figure in a yellow cycling jacket waving frantically at us. As we got closer, I could see that Jane was now even trimmer than she had been only ten days earlier – and with a deeper tan she looked the picture of health. I pulled up alongside her and she opened Steven's door, hugged him, un-strapped him, then lifted him out.

I recced the street for parking spots but with no luck – although I did note that Rob's car with two bikes strapped to the back was immediately outside the hotel; how did he manage that?

I found a multistorey car park a few hundred yards away, and parked up. Laden with bags, I found I was gasping for breath and when my legs buckled beneath me I tripped and hit the floor. I felt weak. But like a newborn foal I stood up gracelessly, wheezed and coughed. Weak, I staggered on.

In the hotel room, a familiar scene greeted me as I dumped the bags on the floor. Various bits of Jane's kit were strewn around the room, clothes were hanging from chairs and over the bath. Jane followed up with Steven.

I stepped straight over to the bed and flopped on to it, laying spread-eagled, my face up, my eyes closed.

'Have you been to the doctor?' Jane asked.

'I'm fine,' I said, coughing. 'It's just a cold.'

'Well,' she said, handing Steven a water bottle, 'you look like shit. Steven says you've been really poorly and grumpy.'

I lifted my head up to look at Steven. 'Thanks, mate,' I said. 'Grass me up, why don't you?'

'Well ... you have,' he said innocently.

What followed from Jane was a lecture on how I needed to look after myself, how I was taking on too much work and how I should get the doctors to organise a chest X-ray.

'Men your age die of pneumonia you know, fit blokes struck down. You need to be careful,' she said.

'Thanks for making me feel so much better,' I said and sat up on to my elbows, determined to prove that I was fine.

After resting for a couple of hours, we headed out to the Cathédral Notre-Dame. Its gothic architecture dominated the landscape for miles. In the evening we headed down to the riverside district to eat out overlooking the Canal du Somme. It was Friday night and the riverside bustled with city life and yet there was none of the intimidation or unpleasant drunkenness that we'd get at home. We ate a beautiful Italian meal and drank lots of water. We chatted and for two blissful hours forgot about The Ride.

Next morning, however, those relaxing two hours were a distant memory as Jane and Luke headed off on a long day's ride to Lille. Originally the plan had been to head directly north to Calais, as the route looked short and undemanding. But conscious that the ride should be a challenge, I prompted Jane to take a late decision and go via Belgium; a slight detour – of 150 miles.

Steven and I headed off to Arras, a town that was preparing for a different cycling occasion a few weeks hence – the Tour de France. I'd hoped to take Steven on a guided tour of the labyrinth of underground passages but Steven squealed at the thought, so we gave it a miss and sat in the Place des Héros and had our dinner.

Afterwards, we got into the car and began our drive to Lille. It would take three hours and the roads were clear so we would reach it in time to see Jane finish. The flat meadows stretched into the distance with just the gentlest of crests occasionally providing opportunities for a good view of the distance.

As we left Arras further behind, the number of cemeteries by the roadside increased. The cemeteries were of varying sizes packed with white-crossed headstones. Each nationality had a different cemetery. We stopped at the Canadian National Memorial at Vimy Ridge and sat for a

303

while reflecting on the loss of so much young life. Steven gripped my hand tighter.

'Are you okay?' I asked.

'Is Mummy going to die soon, Dad?'

I was saddened by the knowledge that despite his mum looking so fit and well her mortality was still in the foreground. 'I don't know,' I said. 'Let's hope not.' I put my hand on his shoulder and we meandered slowly back to the car.

Lille was European Culture Capital which seemed something of a misnomer as it looked like little more than a huge industrial estate dominated by factories and transportation infrastructure. We arrived at the hotel to find Rob already in the prime parking spot and Jane came soon afterwards. There was an air of celebration amongst the cyclists as their average speed had reached 18 m.p.h. – the fastest of the ride so far.

Despite the early finish, it was 7.30 p.m. by the time Jane returned from doing a *Sky News* live spot on the side of the canal and we were all famished. Although our European neighbours think nothing of starting their main meal at ten or even eleven at night, Jane suffers vomiting if she eats too late and so we headed out of the hotel to look for a restaurant.

We entered the thriving Place du Général de Gaulle, which was packed with milling crowds, flags and banners adorning the lampposts. The square was surrounded by narrow streets filled with cafés, shops and restaurants. Tables were at a premium but Luke spotted a free one at an Italian restaurant and we grabbed it.

By the time we'd finished our meal it was 9.30 p.m. but the city's atmosphere was too vibrant to leave for the hotel. We wandered down the rue de Paris to the Place Volint. It was exactly as I'd imagined a cosmopolitan city in continental Europe to be on a Saturday night; loud, brash without the merest whiff of trouble. As Steven tired we headed back to the hotel, promising to return for a weekend in the future.

Within minutes of getting back to the hotel Steven was asleep on the floor in a sleeping bag at the side of our bed. Jane wrote in her diary, which she had placed on her propped-up duvet, while I rubbed her back.

'Just a bit lower,' she said, guiding my fingers with her left hand.

'Are you okay?' I asked. Her face had gone as white as a porcelain pot.

'Yes, it's just from eating late,' she said.

That night, despite my best efforts to stay awake to keep Jane company, I failed to do so. Some hours later, I awoke to find the room illuminated from the cracks in the bathroom door and the sound of Jane vomiting.

I sat up. 'Are you okay?' I called. There was no response. I didn't want to invade her space so I lay silently until she rejoined me. 'That may help,' I said.

'I'm in a lot of pain, Mike. The bottom of my back's very sore.'

'Do you want me to rub it?'

'Life's disappointing enough already,' she said, but ignoring her I started to massage the area.

305

Soon, however, sleep was upon me. I awoke again to the sound of the bathroom tap glugging water. I sat up. The digital alarm blinked 3.10 a.m. Jane walked back in through the bathroom door, her eyes swollen, wiping her face with a flannel. There was no disguising the fact that she had been crying.

'What's up?' I asked, a little alarmed.

'It's my back, Mike. I'm in so much pain.'

'Do you need a doctor?'

'No, I'm going to get a bath to see if I can get rid of some of the spasm. Don't look so worried.' With that, she was off. I lay awake until Jane returned forty minutes later, wrapped in a towel, her face etched with pain. She climbed back into bed and tried to find a position she could tolerate.

Neither of us slept and at six thirty Jane got up and went downstairs. Steven slept on, oblivious, until Jane returned.

'How are you?' I said.

'Dreadful.'

I watched as she changed into her cycling shorts and tops. 'What are you doing?'

'The "live" with Sky.'

'You're joking,' I said, getting out of bed. 'I can do that. You can't cycle today.' I grabbed my jeans and T-shirt. 'You look like shit.'

'Not a word to anyone, Mike. I mean it. I just need to set off.'

I shook my head. 'Jane, you've been up all night being sick ... back pain. Get real. You can't cycle eighty miles. It's preposterous.'

'There's no alternative,' she said. 'I just don't want anyone to know – and definitely not the media. It's my illness, my life. I've told Ian not to ask me how I am or I'll just blank his question.'

The location for the live broadcast was the same as last night – down by the canal and half an hour's drive away so it was some time before she returned. Jane emerged from the hotel having packed the rest of her pannier, no less meticulous because of the pain and the sickness.

'Okay everyone,' she said, chivvying us along. Within minutes they were off on the rain-soaked road to Roubaix. As she pushed her left pedal down there was a determination to her face, her jaw clenched, her mouth tight shut. 'Come on, Luke,' she shouted, and they were gone.

JANE

We were nearing the end of the French leg of our journey. The days on the bike seemed to last longer and longer and we were enjoying more and more the respites at tiny cafés and choco-latiers, knowing they would soon be over.

'We're on the very last map of France and look we're nearly at Calais,' I said to Luke outside one such café.

'It's a good job we're near the end – look at the state of it,' Luke said. The map was laced with holes where it had been folded to fit into the map bag.

The grandeur of Paris had given way to small rural villages. As we passed through the different areas, the architectural style changed consider-ably. Some towns had stone-clad houses, others red herringbone brick.

We bumped along a mean gravel lane, stones clunking under the wheels. 'One day Champs Elysées, the next this,' Luke muttered as we jolted our way along.

'Look at the name of the hotel.' I passed the paper to Luke.

'Grand Hôtel de l'Universe,' he said. 'That doesn't bode well, does it?' Our experience of hotels called 'grand' and 'palace' made us very sceptical of descriptive names. They could be shabby run-down hostelries with lumpy un-comfortable beds.

We arrived in the town centre of Amiens and, unable to orientate ourselves, I stopped at a hotel and asked if they had a map of the area. The concierge duly passed over a small photocopied map and we navigated ourselves to the north of the town, past the grand medieval cathedral that held a maze in its lofty interior.

When we arrived at our hotel – the best hotel in the universe – we were pleasantly surprised to find it was a small well-run establishment and the rooms were very comfortable.

Later in the afternoon I watched anxiously from the small park at the corner of the hotel trying to spot Mike as he drove in. He was a little later than he had expected to be. Finally, we found each other. 'It's been a bloody awful jour-ney,' he said as he dragged his suitcase in one hand, Steven clutching the other.

'Mummy!' Steven cried and I bent to give him a hug. They would be with me for at least a week,

Mike had booked some leave from work so that we could spend some time together, and I had been looking forward to it.

It was our last day in France but before heading to England we planned to cycle over the border to Belgium, to see another part of Europe. We were so close to the border that it seemed too good an opportunity to miss. The only evidence of being in another country, however, was the unfamiliar signage and the different names to the towns.

I had heard about the fabulous Belgian chocolates and cafés, and as we cycled into Ypres the vast grey-cobbled square had cafés all the way around. It was overlooked by the municipal building, tall roofed, with a spire stretching up and tiny windows in the eaves. We sat under an umbrella to shelter from the rain and waited for our coffees.

'We're heading back to the UK,' said Luke. 'I can feel it in my bones.' As we sheltered, many people came up to us curious about the tandem. Some were French, some Belgian but I was surprised by the number of British families holidaying as well.

'You're nearly home, Jane,' said one woman cheerfully.

'Everyone keeps saying that,' I said. 'But we've still got a long way to go, over four hundred miles.'

Leaving Belgium and heading back towards Dunkirk, we kept glancing to our right to try to catch a glimpse of the sea. 'Look,' I said, 'I can see kites but no beach.' Red and yellow kites dived and soared freely beside us as we laboured along the road running parallel to the unseen coast. The petrochemical works at Dunkirk were detectable by their odour before we actually saw them. We'd cycled nearly sixty miles and still had over twenty miles to go to make it into Calais; our last stop in France before we caught the ferry back to England the next day.

'We'll stop here; I need a rest,' Luke said, as we pulled off the main road where an abandoned mattress lay a few yards away. Admiring the view he said, 'I think I might bring the missus here – to one of our impromptu picnic stops.'

I smiled. 'Yes, I think Mike and Steven would enjoy the view too.' Suddenly, I jumped up from the grass, hopping from one leg to another.

'What's that girly noise for?' asked Luke as I squealed and swatted at my legs.

'Ants!' I yelped. 'They're crawling all over my feet!'

We got back on the bike and started pedalling. As we approached Calais, the tarmacked surface in the town was a smooth relief to our bodies after the bone-juddering roads of Belgium. Towards the centre a blue car pulled alongside us.

'It's Jane, isn't it?' said a woman's voice. The car had slowed to our pace and the passenger looked at us. 'Here, let me give you this,' she said and held out a twenty-pound note. It waved in the wind and I put out my hand to grasp it.

'Thank you, that's very kind,' I said as I fumbled to put it in my small bag around my waist. The car sped off and the children in the back craned to wave at us.

'It smells of holidays,' Luke said.

'Yes, Ainsdale beach at Southport.'

'We might see the sea soon.' We both raised ourselves, trying to catch our first glimpse of the shoreline. We pulled up at the front where the sands led down to the water. I put my hands over my brow, shielding my eyes from the glare of the sun, and we sat looking and looking. The heat haze cleared slightly and there before us, miles away, were the white cliffs on the other side of the Channel.

'Look, it's England!' I shouted. I was excited, so long away from home and suddenly there were the white cliffs before me. The heat haze settled again and the shores of England disappeared from view once more.

On our final day in France, everyone was up early to catch the Eurotunnel to Folkestone.

'One, two, three,' Luke said, as he and Mike hoisted the tandem high and manoeuvred it on to the roof bars of the car. It sat there without its front wheel and Luke finished securing it, placing straps tightly around the frame.

Sitting in the car on our way to the Eurotunnel, I couldn't get over how fast we were moving. Our sedate 15 m.p.h. over the last twenty-nine days suddenly seemed bewilderingly slow as fields, lampposts and traffic whizzed by at 60 m.p.h. on the motorway. We passed under the sign 'tunnel sous La Manche' and slowed as we joined the queues.

Leaving France was such a big step. We would be back in England and would feel we were on the final leg of our homeward journey. Standing beside the car in the long silver train, we watched the countryside through the window as it moved by us. All of a sudden the train descended into the tunnel and there was only blackness out of the window.

'Twenty miles today without pedalling,' Mike said. 'Maybe we should take the bike down and have you pedalling as we travel.'

'Get lost,' I said.

At the other end, we followed the cars from the train back into the bright daylight and journeyed to Dover. 'Back in England,' Mike said as we stood outside Pollyanne's fish and chip shop.

'Fish and chip time it is then,' I said as Steven bounced beside me.

'End of cake time, I think,' said Luke. 'That's a shame. I think I preferred cakes to fish and chips.'

MIKE

Sitting on the pebbles of Dover beach, her lycra legs tucked underneath her, Jane was concentrating hard on the questions being asked by an inquisitive journalist. Prior to starting the ride, Jane and I had agreed I'd have carte blanche to arrange as many interviews as possible from Folkestone to Leeds. Nearby, Luke checked the bike's mechanics as he had throughout the journey, ensuring that the short trip on the Euro-tunnel hadn't caused any technical issues. We'd driven back from Folkestone to Dover to avoid the criticism that Jane had not travelled the full distance from Rome to Leeds. It was a preposterous notion – bearing in mind the distance was only twelve miles – but it was better to be safe.

After finishing the interview and posing for some pictures, Jane and Luke set off northwards. Steven and I sauntered into the centre of Dover. The bank holiday heat was pleasant rather than hot. There's a point in every journey where the appearance of familiar landmarks announces that you're nearly there. When travelling to see my folks up in Settle, it was always spotting the sign for Ingleborough. Likewise, when travelling up from London to Leeds on the train, the station at Doncaster was always a comforting sight. For this particular adventure, a small fish and chip shop in Dover meant that Jane was nearly home and the journey would be over for all of us.

After the interview, Steven and I set off to the Travel Inn at Folkestone while Jane, Luke and Martyn began to cycle.

Since arriving in Amiens I'd been feeling increasingly unwell, hot sweats, painful chest and coughing up an unseemly amount of phlegm. I'd pondered whether to stay on the road or go home to rest but on reflection thought I would be more of a liability than help if I stayed. I decided to head home as opposed to staying for the last week of the ride as previously planned. It seemed foolish to waste a week of annual leave to travel with Steven alongside Jane and Luke, when just functioning on a daily basis was becoming impossible.

'What time are you setting off?' These were Jane's first words after alighting from the bike in Folkestone. Her helmet and gloves were soon off;

313

she unzipped the front of her yellow jacket to reveal a trail of mud splashes up the back. Luke wheeled the tandem away, leaving us alone.

'I just need to do an interview, then I'm off,' I said.

'You look ghastly. Are you going to be okay to drive home?'

'Yes.'

'Is it me?' she asked. I'd anticipated that she would ask that question as one of her characteristics is always to think everything's her fault.

'Don't be silly.'

'Are you sure?'

I hugged her, saying, 'I'm not well, it won't be much fun for Steven and it's a waste of a week's holiday we could have together later.' I carried on, 'I'm just ill. No more and no less; I'm worse than I thought. I need to get home and see a doctor.'

We hugged again. Within an hour, Steven and I had gone. Jane looked desolate as we left. A too visible reminder that although the white cliffs had been reached she still had the length of England to ride; a journey in itself.

JANE

I had been distraught that Mike would not be staying with us for the final part of the journey. When I had been unwell, and the pain had been very bad on the bike, the thought that Mike would soon be with me had kept me pedalling. At first, I didn't understand why he wouldn't stay, but finally accepted that he was ill himself, and needed to go home to rest.

After seeing the majestic cliffs of Dover, both Luke and I felt we were truly on our way homewards. The sky in England seemed different somehow, the light much more ... British. As we were only twenty miles or so away from France, it really shouldn't have been so, but the whole countryside had a very English feel.

I reminded Luke that we now had to check to our right rather than our left at the roundabouts after he went into autopilot at the beginning of the ride. We followed the lanes that took in some of the Pilgrim's Way. Along Long Barn Lane, the skeletal fingers of a lightning-struck tree spread out towards us from among the tall hedgerows. Craning our necks, we tried to catch a glimpse round the next corner, listening for any oncoming cars. The sweet echoes of a cuckoo sounded as the rain lessened.

Arriving at Dartford several hours later the rain which had been pouring down for most of the journey eased for a while. Luke and I sat on the wall of a petrol station, steeling ourselves for our journey into London. The traffic grew heavier and heavier as we neared the city. People rushing home from work roared by us, skirting our bike by inches and throwing up spray from their wheels, drenching us further. We pushed our way up Shooter's Hill in south London, through the river of water gushing down it.

'So are you enjoying London?' I said to Luke as we neared the top of the hill and headed for Greenwich.

'It's worse than the Arc de Triomphe,' he

315

shouted back at me. 'What's it like for you?' I shook my head and laughed.

We cycled through the park at Greenwich, enjoying the reprieve from the traffic, and stopped briefly at the *Cutty Sark*, rain dripping from its sail-less mast. Back on the road with the horrendous traffic, at least we could see Big Ben up in the distance as we pushed down the Embankment.

Waiting for us in Westminster, were the *Sky News* team. 'What was that like?' asked Ian Dovaston, the reporter. Luke and I unclasped our helmets stretching our necks.

'Eighty two and a half miles from Folkestone and it's rained all day,' Luke replied. 'We're relieved to be here. We're tired and wet and it's been one of the longest days cycling. And it's now ten to seven by Big Ben's reckoning.'

'I think we need to change out of this gear and eat,' I said. Luke nodded in agreement, looking at me with sunken hollowed eyes.

I had promised Mike that he could organise a media schedule the next day and boy did he make the most of it. With a 6 a.m. start to get to *GMTV* followed by an interview for *Sky News* at Westminster only a few minutes later, Mike was working us hard to get as much publicity as possible and to raise as much money as we could in the last week of the ride.

We finished mid-afternoon and, sitting on a bench, we wearily sipped at a coffee. It had been a long day and we had been interviewed by so many journalists that the interviews all blurred into one.

The day wasn't over though till we had cycled to Isleworth to the Sky News studios. Sky had been with us for the entire journey and wanted to celebrate our return to England. We were to cycle into the studio and be interviewed live.

An hour later we were out of the studio and were heading to Hayes, just an hour's journey away. Back along the Thames there was evidence of the rain and tides. Cars parked too close to the water were now sitting in the river. 'They'll not be pleased,' said Martyn, who had rejoined us to cycle through London and then to Hayes.

We ambled alongside the river for a while before heading towards the busy main road and our hotel stop for the night.

MIKE

Tonight's hotel was on the edge of Glossop. The long gravel drive led up to some parking places which separated the rather grand house from a manicured front lawn.

'I bet they were all like this,' I said, taking a pannier from Jane. Steven and I had driven from Ashbourne – the previous night's stop.

'You've seen the best with Valouse and this one,' she said. 'Some have been incredibly dire.'

I winked at Steven. 'We don't believe you, do we, Steven?'

'No,' said Steven. 'They're all posh.' He grabbed the football from the boot. 'Can we play?'

'Will you shut up, Mike?' said Jane grumpily. 'If you had any idea what it's been like on the road

317

you'd shut up now.' She flung her jacket at me, its toggle hitting the car. All the cyclists were a little tetchy immediately after dismounting until they'd eaten, drank and orientated themselves.

'Calm down, dear, it's only a bike ride,' I said. Jane mouthed a profanity and moved away across the drive where another photographer was waiting. I followed her to brief him that the shoot would last a maximum of ten minutes – after fifteen minutes I returned asking him to make this his last shot. He ignored me, his camera clicking away as Jane posed with the bike.

'Jane,' he said. 'If we could just have you tinkering with the bike, kneel on the gravel, will you, love?'

I stepped forward, my hand out. 'Sorry, pal, that's it,' I said. 'Come on, Jane, we need you inside.'

'Just one more,' he pleaded.

'No,' I said insistently. If every press photographer had their way, Jane would have spent the majority of the ride posing for their publication. Jane took her cue to leave and went inside, leaving the photographer a little disgruntled. I decided to have a kick about with Steven, keeping an eye on the photographer as he packed up.

Our numbers were swollen for the last night with myself, Steven, Cassie from SPARKS and some journalists. We accounted for 90 per cent of the guests and we had to be seated in separate rooms for dinner. Despite being so close to the end of the ride, everyone was aware that there was another fifty miles to go including the renowned

Holme Moss, a notable climb included in all Britain's major cycling races and added here to add some credibility to what Jane was doing; so it wasn't time to celebrate just yet.

At dinner, I leant over to Jane. 'We've got something for you,' I said. 'Steven, do you want to go and get Mum the bag.' Within a minute Steven returned smiling and he handed his mum a carrier bag containing two yellow jerseys.

'It's for tomorrow, Mum. The last stage,' he said, 'but you can't wear them because the lettering's too small.'

'Thank you,' she said, leaning down to give him a kiss. 'I don't ever want to be apart from you again.' She welled up and hugged him tighter. 'Are you coming to the finish?' she asked.

Steven beamed. 'Yes! Grandma's getting me from school at dinnertime.'

'Where *is* the finish, Mike?' Jane asked.

'I don't know, Millennium Square, I guess. There'll just be a couple of us there to welcome you back. Suzanne can't make it; she's got an exam.'

'No police motorcycle outriders this time then?' she said, pulling a cheeky face.

'No – just us. Your mum's going to try and get down as well.'

Jane looked at us and said, 'I'll just be glad to get home.'

JANE

The day started early. We needed to set off at 7

319

a.m. to arrive in Leeds for 1.30 p.m. Ian filmed us as we left and we waved as we sailed down the small lane. Our last start and so near the finish. Martyn was cycling alongside us and was as excited as us. Luke unzipped his top. 'I've got me yellow jersey on,' he said.

I unzipped my top. 'I've got mine on too.' We showed Martyn small glimpses of our yellow tops saved for this last day. The road was quiet, the clouds grey, hanging on to the very peaks we where about to climb. Single cars passed us widely, then roared on. At the bottom of the climb we passed Torside Reservoir and then the road steepened.

'We're about to do Holme Moss,' Martyn said, 'which is a good Pennine climb.' He added, 'Hopefully after Mont Ventoux this should be a breeze.' Our legs, strong from so many days' cycling, pushed round and round. The adrenalin of the prospect of actually reaching our home town pushing us faster and faster. The gradient grew cruelly steeper and we were puffing now.

'Can you see that mast? There, that's the top,' I said to Luke, and it drew us up. We crawled up the road, cycling alongside the white kerbside marker. On and on, the top beckoning us as the clouds seemed to lower to sit on the very hillside we were cycling up.

'Are we classed as cycling fit now?' Luke asked.

'I dunno. It's quite hard, isn't it?' The roadside markers passed by, the crash barriers towards the top striped black and white. We soared to the top and, lightly pedalling, we felt the blood circulating and our muscles relaxing once more.

'Have you seen that?' Luke asked, indicating a banner at the side of the road. It had balloons waving from it, 'WELCOME HOME' in large letters at the top and bottom and between them the words 'YORKSHIRE BORDER CONTROL AHEAD PLEASE HAVE YOUR PASSPORTS READY FOR INSPECTION.'

Martyn had cycled all the way from Rome with us. Every turn of the pedals had been his as well. 'It's my mum and dad,' he said. 'We're back in Yorkshire.' I nodded at him and the bubbling inside me at being home was nearly too much to control. 'It feels like home,' he babbled. 'I'm a Yorkshire lad following a Yorkshire lass and it feels great.' We fell from our bikes and clasped cold hands round warm cups of coffee from flasks from Martyn's parents.

Our schedule saw us soon back on the bikes continuing our journey. Downhill we quickly ended up in Huddersfield. A small hill out of Flockton surprised us and as Luke knocked down the gears we slowly crept up the steep incline. 'I think I'm sweating more than up Ventoux,' Martyn said.

'That's probably due to your cake consumption since Ventoux,' I retorted. As we passed through the small Yorkshire towns people stood on the roadside, waiting to see us cycle by. Clapping us on, roaring at us. One woman dashed from her kitchen waving her teatowel as a flag at us.

Our legs seemed light and the bike sped along. Our high spirits making it seem like some young black stallion as we sailed through Wakefield and then along to Rothwell. The hairs on the back of my neck crept up as we passed the stone sign showing us we were entering my home village. 'Can we go to see Steven at his school?' I asked. 'Mike said we might try to get there.'

'If you want,' Luke said, as we turned left at the end of the road and pulled into Steven's primary school. Pushing the bike into the playground we were soon lost in a crowd of youngsters. Steven stood at my side looking up at me.

'Come on, come on,' Mrs Reynolds called. 'Let's line up and give Luke and Jane a big welcome.'

'Three cheers!' The cries echoed around the yard.

'Where's Martyn?' I asked Luke.

'I think he's still round the front,' he said.

'There's one important person missing,' I called and dashed round to find Martyn. Sat on the pavement, he stood and followed me round and as we sat in the semicircle of children Mrs Reynolds called, 'Three cheers for Martyn.' More cries rang out from their lips.

'You almost looked like you were going to cry,' I said to Martyn when the echo of the cheers had died away.

'I've never had cheers like that before,' he replied. 'I've seen you get them but those were just for me.' His face split with a grin, his eyebrows raised.

We set off for the city, passing landmarks we had missed for the last five weeks. The City Square with its Black Prince could have easily been in any

322

European city. Then we were heading up Park Row towards our final destination in front of the City Art Gallery. We stopped at the traffic lights and could see the crowds lining either side of the road, several people deep on to the Square. Then we were only a few pedal strokes from the finish. The crowds were shouting, people applauding loudly their arms raised; there were cheers and whistles and shouts of 'Well done.' Balloons waved from the hands of children standing behind barriers. The wheels of the bike rolled over the letters in white across the Square. HOME it said and we were home.

Ian from Sky was once more with us. He had seen us set off in Rome and here we were 1900 miles later. 'We've made it all the way from Rome,' I said and patted Luke on the bike. 'Thank you, Luke. It's been really difficult.' My lips quivered. I knew the tears streaming from my eyes would be unseen.

'It's been a fantastic adventure for Jane and me and Martyn who has travelled with us,' Luke said. 'It's been a fabulous adventure but extremely hard work and we're glad just to have made it home safely.' Over £150,000 had been raised since we'd set off – more than we could ever have imagined. We finally climbed from the bike and the applause started and didn't stop; cheers and whistles carried on for long long minutes.

CHAPTER 9

June 2004

MIKE

Jane hadn't settled since she'd returned home. Although we'd metaphorically shut the front door behind us when she and Luke had finished the ride, we'd not really managed to isolate ourselves as much as we'd wanted. Thousands of letters from supporters were piling up in the front room, covering every available work surface and remaining unanswered. Every time I looked at the growing pile, it pricked my conscience and made me miserable. The response from the public had been beyond any of our hopes. I was beginning to feel overwhelmed by everything and couldn't see a finish. Still, we had a holiday to Lake Garda to look forward to. Rebecca's exams were drawing to a conclusion and we were due to drive on the day after her last one.

It was lunchtime Wednesday and I'd just nipped out to the building society to update the passbooks on Jane's charity account. Incredibly, over £200,000 had been deposited in the account in the last seven days and the young cashier behind the counter couldn't quite believe what she was seeing. Page after page was filled with lines of fresh data – we managed to fill three books in total and I overran my lunch break by fifteen minutes.

Back at the office, I put the passbooks in my back pocket and noticed a scrap of paper on the keyboard of my laptop asking me to call Jane urgently. I checked my mobile and noticed a missed call and so picked up my phone. Jane answered almost immediately.

'Mike, you need to come home.' There was a hint of alarm in her voice.

'What's up?'

'I've had a threatening phone call.' I relaxed slightly. There'd been a number of them, all from cranks, which had amounted to little more than a nuisance.

'Another? That's the third since you've come home.'

'Not abusive. Threatening.'

'How so? What did he/she say?'

'That he was going to come down and do me in.'

Despite the seriousness of the call, it was hard not to raise a smile. 'Well, he can fuck off and go to the back of the queue,' I said. 'I hope you told him.'

Jane sighed. 'Well, I'm glad you find it funny.' I pressed the keys to unlock my screen. 'Are you typing?'

'No.'

'The number wasn't withheld – should I ring the police?'

'Well, let's have the number and see where he comes from first,' I said, grabbing a pen while Jane reeled off a landline number.

I scribbled it down. 'Listen, I'll come home if you want me to but I don't think we should worry about anything prematurely – let's do some digging and just see where we are first.'

'I'm really scared, Mike. I know you think it's funny but it wouldn't be funny if you were sat here with me.'

Within five minutes we'd tracked down the caller to a Scottish isle, ten minutes later we had a name and address. It was clear to us that even if the gentleman actually wanted to attack Jane, there was little he could do about it from where he was. By the evening we'd decided not to contact the police but to go ex-directory and change our number when we got back from Italy.

During the weeks following Jane's return, we received dozens of requests from the media, asking Jane – or occasionally myself – to be interviewed. One young researcher even asked if I would go on BBC radio to comment on Tony Blair's proposed educational reforms. The devil in me considered it for a few seconds but in the end I politely declined and told her that Mike Tomlinson, the former Chief Inspector of Schools, was in a much better position than me to share his thoughts. In fact, we turned down all the media requests. As a family – and as a couple – we were desperate to restore some semblance of normal life and the only way we could do that was to shun any kind of publicity. Jane had returned to work and that in itself was comforting to her – it gave her a sense of routine that I think she'd missed.

After persistent nagging from Jane that I should

see someone about my cough, I agreed to let her come to the doctor's with me. My chest had felt as though I was carrying a lead weight so Jane was convinced I had pneumonia; she wasn't wrong. I'd been signed off work for two weeks and the chest X-ray had proved that rest had resolved most of the acute symptoms, although the consultant said it could take up to four months to get back to normal.

It was ironic that Jane had been preaching to me about my own health care while she was struggling to make a decision about having radiotherapy. I could understand her dilemma. While the treatment would alleviate some of the pain in her bones, there was no doubt that it might damage her internal organs. It was a decision she would have to make herself but I couldn't help noticing how the pain was severely limiting her life.

One Saturday afternoon having just parked up to get some last-minute shopping for our holidays, she hobbled down the stairs of the multistorey car park at Woodhouse Lane; there was no disguising her discomfort. I offered to take her grey rucksack. She stopped, dipped her left shoulder and let the bag slide off. It was ridiculously heavy.

'What the fuck's in 'ere?' I said, as the strap of the bag dug into the skin of my hand.

'Bits,' Jane said, setting off down the road.

'Bits? No wonder your shoulder hurts, hod carriers lift less weight than this. We're only getting some holiday clothes, why did you need to bring this into town.'

She stopped and looked at me, holding out her

327

arm. 'If you're gonna moan, hand it back.'

I ignored her and carried on walking. We dodged the traffic at the lights and headed down Woodhouse Lane towards Albion Street, one of the main arterial roads into town.

'Have you decided what to do about having some radiotherapy?' I asked tentatively. I'd noticed that Jane had been taking regular doses of stronger painkillers. Her constant checking of the time to ensure that the day's next dose could be taken at the first opportunity was a dead giveaway of her declining health.

'No,' she said.

We proceeded to the top of Albion Street where the crowds of shoppers were increasing in density; bus stops overflowed, partially blocking the pavement.

'What about the triathlon have you made a decision yet to compete or not?' The triathlon was seven days after we returned from holiday, so it was imperative that she made her decision before we went away in ten days' time.

'No,' she said.

'If you're going to do it you'll need to start training.'

'Oh, shut up. It's a sprint triathlon and if I can't manage that after 2000 miles cycling and a marathon there's something wrong with me.'

'So you *are* doing it, then?'

'Don't you listen? I don't know.'

'Well, what about the ironman?'

'Will you stop mithering me! I don't know what I'm going to do. I'm fed up with the media. My pelvis is so painful I'm struggling to walk, let alone run. I'm tired. I just want it all to stop and you...' Jane turned to face me, the tears were streaming down her face. We stood motionless. Albion Street was packed, although it may as well have been empty as the intensity of our emotions cocooned us.

'What about me?'

'I feel like I'm dying; I can't do any more.' I moved to hug her. 'Just go away, leave me alone.' The tears were flooding down.

As we stood, stranded in the street, a middle-aged woman came up to us, laden with shopping bags. 'It's Jane isn't it? It is! It's Jane, isn't it?' she said.

Jane turned her head away, wiping her tears with her sleeve. 'Yes,' she muffled.

'Oh, I've so wanted to meet you,' said the lady.

Jane shook her hand and moved off abruptly, leaving the lady standing as if in a state of suspended animation. 'I can't deal with this madness any more.'

JANE

The exhilaration of returning to Leeds was short-lived. The pain in my back and down my leg was too great to ignore. I could no longer sleep through it. When I looked in the mirror, even the sun-kissed tan from the many days' cycling couldn't disguise the greyness of my complexion. I was offered radiotherapy on my pelvis to ease the symptoms and, after careful consideration, I eventually decided to opt for it, hoping that it would work.

I hadn't fully appreciated the tiredness I would experience after such a long ride and the purging effect it would have on my insides. After just a day, the discomfort of my pain was replaced by terrible stomach cramps and flu-like listlessness. As the side effects subsided I knew the decision to have radiotherapy had been the right one. For the first time in weeks I could lie down without pads and pillows placed around me to support my back and hips. I slept through the night and woke feeling refreshed. I could look forward to the family holiday in Italy at Lake Garda.

Sitting on sun loungers placed on the sparse grass at the campsite, Mike and I could finally fully relax. Away from any distractions, family life slowed down to holiday pace, and it was only Steven who still moved at full pelt – racing around the small area outside the static caravan.

The pool was noisy with children splashing and ducking, diving and bombing but one lane was set aside for swimming. Rebecca and I were in the lane, trying to get in some much needed training for the Salford Triathlon which Rebecca, Suzanne and I were due to take part in on the return from our holiday. With the cycle trip and then the radiotherapy, I hadn't been able to go to the International Pool as I would have done normally.

Each day while we were away I tried to run a little further but although the radiotherapy had eased my pain it had left me exhausted and I tired easily. It made my running heavy and ungainly. Rebecca ran with me and was a great encouragement. Each night I forced myself to run along the lakeside, plodding slowly in the low sunshine. The air still warm from the heat of the day, I would return to the caravan to wash the salty sweat from my body under the cool dribble of water from the shower head.

Mike and I would then sit outside and watch Steven playing football with other young lads on the campsite. They were many nationalities, including Danish, Belgian and Irish, but they didn't need language to communicate.

We returned home from our break a day early to allow us to unpack and then repack to go to Salford to take part in the triathlon. Suzanne, Rebecca and I set off on the Sunday morning under a squally sky. We cajoled each other round the run course. Suzanne cramped up at the beginning and then Rebecca and then me. We had a slow time of it but the collective experience of running over the bridge towards the finish was worth it.

After tea back home, I managed to clear the kitchen and tried busily to catch up with my friends and family after being away for three weeks. I phoned my friend Michelle who was panicking about getting her packing finished for her summer holidays. I phoned my brother Mark whose daughter had been unwell. I put the phone down and picked it up again to call Jackie. I could hear the intermittent dialling tone that told me a message had been left. I dialled 1571.

'You have two new messages.' The first new message: 'If you don't stop coming on the tele-

331

vision...' It was a woman's angry voice – at first I thought it was one of my friends trying to wind me up, but then I listened more. 'If you don't stop coming on the television as a fucking charlatan you'll hear from my solicitor. You're nothing but a fucking fraud.'

Her s's were hissed sibilants, her f's furiously pronounced. I saved the message and listened to the next. The same woman's voice abused me. This time her voice was even angrier, her spitefulness clear in her murderous tones. 'Why don't you do us all a favour and fucking die? Then we don't have to listen to your pathetic lies.'

I was gripping the handset tightly by now. 'Mike, you need to listen to this,' I said.

Mike came and took the phone from me and listened, his eyes widening with surprise. 'Don't pay any attention,' he said. 'She's obviously off her trolley.'

Suzanne appeared at the top of the stairs. 'Is it that woman again?' she asked.

'Well it's some mad bitch,' I said. 'Why? Has she rung before?'

Suzanne nodded. 'Yes, while you were away. I didn't know what to do. She was so nasty I didn't get a chance to say anything. She just said some horrible things and then put the phone down. Cynthia came and sat with me because I was so upset.'

'Bloody hell, Mike,' I said. 'I'm not letting her get away with that. At least let's get the number changed.'

I picked up the phone to try to speak to the operator. There was another new message. The woman was sobbing and crying down the phone, sounding like a maudlin drunk. 'Is that Jane Tomlinson?' she sobbed, drawling out my name. 'You're a lying bloody fucking bitch. I've been ringing you all night. I'm dying from breast cancer and you're a lying little lying little lying cow. You're not dying. You're just a fucking bastard liar.' She sobbed into the phone, her voice becoming more slurred. 'If you were terminally ill you'd have been dead by now. You're just a lying cow and you're not on the phone. I've been ringing you since six o'clock.' Her voice started to rise until she was screaming down the phone. 'You're a fucking bastard fucking bastard and I'm going to see you in hospital, you bitch.'

'Bloody hell,' I said. 'She's got herself a bit worked up now.'

Mike took the receiver from me and listened himself. 'I'm not having this,' he said. 'I'm ringing the police. She can't go around doing that.'

The stranger's vehemence was very disturbing and I felt sick that she had subjected myself and my family to her cruel thoughts. I was sure she had obtained our phone number from the telephone book, so she would know my address as well. I worried that she might arrive at my house to confront me. Even worse, she might speak to my children. I was tearful in the moments after listening to her voice.

As the night drew on, the fear turned to anger, and I wanted the chance to show her she couldn't frighten me with her threats. All summer I had been in two minds about the ironman triathlon. Should I go for it? Would I cope with any more public fundraising? Had I the stomach for any more challenges? The woman's malevolence fired me up. If she didn't want to see me on her television she had a clear choice. She could turn the television off.

There was a strange car outside my house when I returned from work the next day. My stomach turned, and I strode up the hill, trying to look into the car to see who might be calling. I let out a long sigh when the car door opened and a female police officer stepped out, hat in hand. 'Jane Tomlinson?' she asked, and I nodded.

'Is it about the phone calls?' I asked.

'Yes, can my colleague and I come in and chat?'

'Yes, of course.' I walked up the drive and unlocked the door, holding it open for the two officers, who stepped through with me into the living room.

'We usually advise people to change their numbers,' the older woman said. 'What did she say to you?'

'You can listen to the messages, if you like. I've saved them on my phone.' They listened and opened their mouths as if to speak, then closed them and listened to the last message.

'Is that a threat she's making?' the younger woman said.

'I don't know, her speech is too slurred by the end.'

'Listen,' said the older woman, 'we'll take the times of the calls and if you can give us permission to look at your phone records we should be able to identify which number called at these times, then we can trace whoever this is.' I nodded. 'We'll go round and have a word with her. It's not on really.'

'I'm more concerned that she's upset one of my children who had to listen to that unpleasantness,' I said. 'The mad cow – she can't do that to us.'

'No, you're right. She might think differently once she's had a visit from us.'

I showed the two women to the door. 'What do I need to do now?' I asked.

'Nothing really, it'll take a few days to sort everything out. We'll be in touch when we've brought her in to talk to her.'

I nodded. 'Well, thanks. It's something and nothing but I'm fed up with people thinking its okay to do this sort of thing.'

'Mum hasn't told them you're coming up,' Mike said as he hauled the bike into the back of the car. 'It should be good training for the triathlon at Nice. You need some hills in your legs.'

'How did I manage to let myself get talked into this?' I asked Mike as we drove into town. It was the last week of the summer holidays. Steven and Rebecca were spending a few days with their grandma in the Dales and I was planning to cycle up to Settle to see them. 'If memory serves me right, the hills out of Nice are more like sheer cliffs,' I said.

My breath caught in my throat in panic just thinking about the climbs out of the town that I would have to cope with if I was to complete the Nice Triathlon. Mark Hayward, who we'd met through his PR for triathlons, had introduced us to his business partner Ryan Bowd. Ryan had suggested that the Nice event would be the perfect warm-up for the Florida triathlon. As he'd offered to accompany me round the course in Nice and in Florida, I wanted to take his advice seriously.

We continued on our journey into Leeds in silence. It was 8.15 a.m. and we'd set off this early to avoid the awful rush hour traffic that made cycling across Leeds difficult and dangerous. It wasn't the miles I needed in my legs, it was the hills more than anything. The strength and stamina not just for my body, but for my mind as well.

I set off on the roads that lead out of Leeds city centre through Headingley out towards Otley and then cycled the quieter back roads along the river towards Ilkley. Bright sunshine was followed by quick, thorough wettings as clouds darkened the sky.

I swung away from Ilkley and headed towards Bolton Abbey. I pushed open the gate that led into the next field and slid myself and the bike through the gap. I could hear a dog barking in the distance, the cows on the brow of the hill looked down at me with interest.

At last I could see a cattle grid in the distance. I gripped the brake lever with my left hand and feathered the right-hand brake lever gently, slowing the bike as I neared the metal bars across the road. Slowed, I bumped safely across them. Looking back at the cattle who were still gently nosing their way towards me I felt relieved to have the grid between myself and the great bovine beasts.

It was great to be cycling again. I'd found the Salford Triathlon hard and hadn't particularly relished being back on the bike, but I'd enjoyed the recent London Triathlon when I had felt stronger. The pain in my back had needed five more sessions of radiotherapy and that had left me exhausted. Now that my body was feeling physically stronger, the muscles in my legs remembered how to meet the challenge of the hills.

The last three miles were swiftly over with. The harsh downhill into Settle required no more effort than hitting heavily on the brake levers all the way down to stop the bike accelerating into blind stone-wall corners.

At the house, I removed my helmet, stretched my neck and knocked on Alice's door. 'Hello,' she said, smiling as she opened it. 'Good cycle?'

'Mummy! Mummy!' Steven leapt up and hugged my legs tightly. 'Uughh, you're all sweaty,' he said.

'What are you doing here?' Rebecca asked.

'I've just cycled from Leeds.'

'What really?' Rebecca exclaimed.

'Yes, really. I'm coming home with you lot when Dad comes up to collect you.'

'Are you going to get a wash or something?' Rebecca stood with her arms folded.

'Get you,' I said. 'Yes, I've even got some clean underwear with me.' I reached into my bag and brought out a sandwich bag with clean smalls in it.

'Mum!' Rebecca said, screwing up her face.

I felt cleaner after my wash despite having to put my dirty and sweaty cycling clothes back on, but at least I had washed the muck from the road from me. I was sitting reading some pages of *Harry Potter* with Steven when Mike arrived.

'Hi, everybody,' he said in a loud jolly voice as he parked his bottom in the spacious armchair. 'Good cycle?'

'Yes, very good thanks. I didn't like the hill into Settle – it was a bit greasy from the rain.'

'I've had a phone call from a woman called Sara from the BBC,' Mike said.

'What was that about?'

'About the documentary you said you didn't want to take part in.'

'Yes and...'

'Well, she'd like to come and visit us the week after next and explain what she'd like to do and listen to anything we might have to say.'

'Oh, right. But she knows we don't want to do it, doesn't she?'

'Well, yes, she knows you're not bothered,' Mike replied. 'Anyway I've said Wednesday night would be okay.'

I let out a large sigh, exasperated at constantly having my life organised for me.

'You've not got anything else planned?' Mike asked.

'Me? What would I be doing?'

'Well, that's all right then, isn't it?'

Sara called at our house the next week. I was confident that nothing would come of the meeting so I was relaxed and sat opposite Sara, sipping at a coffee, ready to listen to her and any proposals she had.

'So what are your plans?' Sara asked. She was very quiet and had listened to all the things Mike had told her that we would not do. We weren't wanting someone to come to film our home lives. If they were going to make a documentary then it should be about an event not our personal family time. 'That all seems 'reasonable,' she said, shifting slightly on the chair and looking at the book she was making notes in. 'It's Nice first and then if everything's fine with Jane you're off to Florida?' she asked. 'And that's November and that's for the ironman?'

I nodded. 'Wow, that's something else,' Sara said. 'I'd be really interested in filming you on that journey. We'd want to film bits of your life but mostly what it's like to train and take part in that sort of event.'

Mike stood and collected the coffee cups from the table. 'So you're off to Nice next weekend?' she said.

I nodded. 'We booked the flights last week. I'm not sure how sensible it is but I really want to complete the ironman this year and I need to know if I can swim the four kilometres. So Nice will be good experience.'

Sara leant forwards in her chair and looked at me directly. 'If I'm going to do this film, I really need to come to Nice,' she said. 'Do you think that would be okay?'

Mike had walked back into the room. 'If you want to come that's fine,' he said. I looked at him, narrowing my eyes and breathing out noisily, cross that yet again he was making decisions for me.

Oblivious, Sara continued. 'I'll have to speak to some people back at the BBC but they're really keen to do this film and I can't see any problems. I'll just have to bring one other person with me. If I get who I've got in mind she's another Sarah as well.'

I was surprised that what had been a chat about proposals was already moving towards actual filming taking place and within a week or so. I looked at Mike as he handed over our flight and hotel details, wondering when he was going to talk to me about what looked like a documentary crew following us over the next month if I was to take part in the Florida Ironman.

Sara shook hands with us as she left. 'I'll ring you tomorrow but I'm pretty sure I'll be coming.'

'We'll look forward to seeing you,' Mike said.

MIKE

The Ibis hotel on avenue Thiers in Nice was functional rather than grand. We'd arrived Friday lunchtime, but when we awoke on Saturday morning, with the triathlon a full twenty-four hours away, rather than rest Jane wanted to go for a swim in the sea, having never done a saltwater swim in a race before. We met the two Sarahs from the BBC in the reception of the hotel. I was surprised to see that the beach was pebbled. Dave and Tony, the cameramen from Yorkshire Television, were already there setting up.

340

The sea was so rough that getting in and out was hazardous. I watched as time after time unsuspecting swimmers were floored by waves that would catch them from behind, sending them to their knees or chins.

'I'm only going to the nearest buoy,' Jane said. I looked out to sea – the nearest orange buoy was bobbing up and down in the choppy waters about 200 yards out.

'This is madness,' I said to our friend Mick, who had accompanied us to Nice to support Jane.

'I guess she knows what she's doing,' he said.

My eyes followed Jane for the first fifty yards until I was confident that she was okay and became distracted by Dave Harrison from Yorkshire Television asking me what we were doing for the rest of the day. When I finally looked out to the water again it was impossible to distinguish Jane from the other swimmers – but what *was* clear, there being no swimmers at all between the shoreline and the buoy, was that she'd already gone further than she'd promised.

'What the fuck is she doing?' I said. All eyes turned out to the sea.

'Can you see her?' I asked Mick. He shook his head.

'Tony can you see her?' Tony was looking through the viewfinder of the camera.

'No,' he said. 'Do you want to have a look, Mike? Will you recognise the stroke or the wetsuit?'

I put my eye to the viewfinder but at that distance there was absolutely no way I would spot her. I moved away muttering to myself about

Jane's recklessness. Steven was sitting on the pebbles talking to a Frenchman, whose dishevelled appearance and deep suntan made me think his nightly accommodation was less than a stone's throw away.

'Steven,' I called and he nonchalantly came over. 'Will you look for Mum?'

'I can't see her,' he said, without even pausing to look.

'Keep trying,' I said.

'What's the problem, Mike?' Dave said.

'There's no safety out there. If she fractures her shoulder in that sea she'll drown.'

'What's the chance of that happening though?' he said.

'It's where the cancer is quite acute – so much greater than you or I.'

In the corner of my eye I saw one of the two Sarahs – Sara Hardy – move her camera closer while Sarah Webster moved her boom mike overhead. 'It's probably not a good time now, Sara,' I said and, to her credit, she moved away instantly. The nomadic Frenchman moved closer in, speaking to Mick while Steven looked through Tony's camera. We stood for an inordinate amount of time, nervously waiting for a glimpse of Jane. Eventually, I spotted her emerging from the water, stumbling forward as the waves hit her back.

I marched down to meet her. Conscious that I was still 'miked up' by the BBC and remembering a recent anecdote of Sarah's about the number of people being caught out on that front, I reached into my back pocket and turned the microphone off. To be doubly sure, I unplugged the wires.

'Hiya,' she said a little breathlessly, shaking off her goggles and smiling. 'Are you all right?' she asked.

'How fucking irresponsible was that?' I barked.

Jane raised her eyebrows at me before walking off towards the others. 'Get over it, Mike,' she said.

'No,' I said, surprised by my own angry tone. 'I won't get–' but she continued marching up the beach and I was left standing there, seething. I knew it wasn't the time to have a stand-up row in front of the others but I swore that I would be having words when we got back to the hotel room.

JANE

I tried to sleep but the memory of the crashing waves on the beach kept me awake. I rose early and dressed as quietly as I could so as not to disturb Steven, who was wrapped cosily in his sleeping bag, his eyes fluttering with dreams. I grabbed my bag and opened the door to leave.

'We'll see you down there,' Mike muttered from underneath the covers. 'Good luck,' he murmured. 'You'll be fine.'

Ryan and the two Sarahs were already in the lobby waiting for me and we headed down the escalator and into the street below. Nice was just starting to come to life. The sun had not yet appeared and the staff at the outdoor cafés were just putting out their chairs and tables, ready for the morning coffee rush. The waves lapped against the stones, no longer churning them up. There was less energy in the sea, it was calmer.

We stood huddled amongst the other triathletes. A race director was giving last minute details in French over a loudspeaker. I couldn't understand any of his words but looked out to the sea and spotted red buoys bobbing out into the distance. My stomach churned and I tasted acid in my mouth as my nerves caused the breakfast to rise in my throat.

'How are you?' Ryan asked. I shook my head, unable to speak, and turned from him as tears of fear ran down my face. My fingers felt numb, my legs too weak to swim for two hours. He put his arm around my shoulder. 'You'll be fine.'

I turned to him. 'Bloody hell, I'm frightened. It's so far out.'

Ryan's grip around my shoulder tightened reassuringly. 'Just watch my cap and I'll keep yelling at you,' he said. 'You can do this.'

A siren sounded and everyone ran towards the water. Splashing through the shallows we moved towards the deeper cooler waters to start swimming. Ryan swam alongside me. I could see him as I turned my head with each breath and I tried to keep up with him. The panic I'd felt before the start was as strong as ever and was making me breathless. I started to push my arms into a breaststroke.

'Crawl, Jane, crawl!' Ryan yelled and so I lifted my arms out of the water to keep up the stroke. We carried on out to sea, passing red buoy after red buoy. The main pack of swimmers drew ever more distant. The waves were large and each dip brought solitude. At each crest, the buoys and Ryan were back in view and if I turned I could make out the lights on the shore at the transition area.

I tugged at my neck and tried to release the Velcro fastening. The hooks were not caught in the fastenings properly and each time my arms passed over my head they rasped against my neck, making it sore. I rubbed my free hand against my neck, treading water for an instant. Ryan turned once more. 'Crawl, Jane, crawl.' I blew out a mouthful of sea water and turned my face into the salty water once more.

At last we reached the shore. I could feel the stones beneath my feet and struggled up the shallows towards the carpeted area of the beach. Somebody hauled me from the water and I stood dazed for a few seconds before heading to the gates in transition.

'Five minutes, Jane, or else we'll not get out the gates,' Ryan yelled at me. I nodded slowly and resumed pulling on my cycling shorts. I smeared sun cream on my arms and neck. The back of my neck, where the skin had rubbed away in the swim, stung, making me yelp.

'Come on!' Ryan urged. I thrust my foot into my shoe and ran with my bike to the gate. We cycled along the flat promenade and Ryan was silent at first. 'I'm sorry about the swim,' he said. 'I think I was sighting someone's swim cap up ahead. It was hard to tell with the swell.'

'Oh, don't worry, at least we made it out of the

water in time.'

We turned right to the hills that stood cliff-like looming over Nice. I could see cyclists ahead of me but as we hit the climbs, the distance from them became stretched as their legs took them away from me. Panting and forcing myself round each bend, up each incline, I swore at the hills, cursing the black tarmac that bounced the heat of the day back at my legs, face and arms.

'I hate you for this, Ryan,' I hissed.

'Come on! You'll thank me later,' he said and I grunted and looked behind me at the car slowly revving at my rear. I lost my balance and nearly collided with the cliff side on my right as I tried to glance at the sign above the motor. In red neon letters were the words 'Finis de Course', confirming what I already thought. That I was indeed the very last cyclist on the road.

'Listen, we'll not make the cut if we don't really push up this next hill,' Ryan said. I nodded. I was already struggling with the incline.

'Bloody hill,' I spat out and it felt good to take my frustration out on the black surface. 'Bloody road,' I roared and I could hear the people in the car behind me chuckling. On and on, the hill rose and we crested it just in time to stop us being disqualified.

The car resumed its slow journey behind me as we started the final climb of the day. We pushed on and on once more. Ryan kept on looking back at the car just behind me until we came to one hairpin and ground round it. Ryan came to a halt and I stopped behind him.

'I don't think they're going to let us continue,'

346

he said. At that, I burst into tears of anger and frustration and pain. Still miles from the finish, I was stuck here unable to carry on.

The small Frenchman stopped his car and came towards us. He shook his head and drew his face down into comic sadness. I shook my head confused. 'C'est complète?' he asked.

'Non,' I replied. I looked up the road 'Continue?'

He nodded his head enthusiastically. 'Ah, oui, continue.' He watched as I mounted my bike and shouted 'Courage' after me as Ryan and I once more set off.

We chased up the rest of the hill and down. My legs circling madly, desperate to retrieve some lost minutes so that we would make the strict time limit for the bike-to-run transition. We could see Nice ahead of us as we started a fast descent down a wide empty road.

Sweeping down, and pedalling on, we crouched low to reduce resistance against the wind and shaved just a few seconds off my time. The last bend was broad and we swept round it now with the transition in view. But just as we could see it clearly we could make out the gate being pulled shut, closing off our entry into transition.

'No!' Ryan cried out, echoing my own silent thought.

MIKE

The number of cyclists returning to the transition area and changing into their running gear had reduced to barely a trickle. The once practically empty area was now full of bikes. For the last two hours, we'd listened as Sara who was following Jane on a media motorbike had provided progress reports on Jane's attempt to defeat the bike/run cutoff time. Her last phone call had been ten minutes ago and she had reported that Jane was eating up the road and would be with us soon.

Dave, Tony the cameraman, and Lia, the journalist from the Press Association, headed off down the road to position themselves ready for Jane's imminent return. Mick, Steven and I stood silently peering down the road for Jane. There was still no sign.

'Dad,' said Steven, suddenly pulling on my sleeve. 'What's the man doing?'

'Where?' I said as Steven pointed in front of us to where two race officials were inching shut the metal gates which would block any more competitors from entering the transition area. A heavily tanned man, wearing a black sleeveless jacket, stood stock still in the middle of the road, staring out into the distance, a mobile phone pressed to his ear.

'I don't know, Steven,' I said as the man placed his phone into his trouser pocket and in a self-important and exaggerated movement made a cross with both arms in front of his chest. A flurry of activity ensued as the two race officials grabbed six-foot high metal barriers from the side of the road, scraping them across the tarmac to seal the transition. I looked at my watch. It was precisely 2 p.m.

'Jane's been timed out,' I said to Mick. He

stood silently, looking down the road to see if there was any sign of her.

'What's happening, Daddy?' Steven asked.

'Mum's been disqualified, Steven. She won't be able to do the run.'

'Oh.' His face dropped.

'Don't worry, at least we'll be able to get back to the hotel early.'

'Yippee.'

Seconds later, Jane and Ryan appeared, their heads down, their legs pushing as hard as possible. Unaware of the impending problem at the transition area, I saw the three camera crews filming Jane as she sped past them. I watched, helpless from behind the metal security barriers at the side of the road, as Jane approached the closed transition area and like a reveller being barred from a nightclub, I saw her being prevented from racing any further. My heart went out to her. The officious man in black grabbed her handlebars, signalling for her to dismount, then, in what I thought was an appalling show of overzealousness, he detached the competitor number from her chest and ripped it in two.

Jane dissolved into a flood of tears. Eight long hours of effort to be cut off by a mere ninety seconds. She was inconsolable and crumpled in front of us. I just wanted to go over to her, to put my arm around her but couldn't get past security.

Lia appeared like a genie out of a bottle. 'I can't believe what they've done, how pathetic. Typical French officialdom, they must have known it was Jane and she was about to finish.'

I shrugged. 'Rules are rules. You know, Lia, if they bend the rules for Jane, where does it stop? She competes as an equal. If she succeeds then it's a proper victory. If they'd let her continue, it would mean nothing.'

'It's not right though,' Lia said.

'It is. When Jane finishes the ironman, it'll be because she deserves to – not as a favour because she's dying. Yes, it's pathetic what they've done, but it's proper – the success will be sweeter when it comes.'

With her number ceremoniously removed, Jane was allowed to re-enter transition to collect her kit bags. She cut a solitary sad and desolate figure. Steven, Mick and I could do little except watch forlornly from a distance until she'd meticulously collected everything.

In fact, I'd been praying that Jane would be timed out. The point of going to France was for Jane to do a difficult sea swim and then have a go at the most difficult bike course in Europe. Florida would be much easier than this; she'd be six weeks fitter. The effort involved in trailing an exhausted body over the run course could mean that her body wouldn't recover in time to compete in a full ironman.

Jane was disconsolate throughout the afternoon. Although we tried to raise her spirits, praising her extraordinary efforts, she was unable to rise above the gloom. In her eyes, she had been disqualified and couldn't see any achievement despite having completed the swim and the ride.

That evening all ten of us headed out to the Place Garibaldi, where we sat outside eating pizza and sharing a bottle of red wine. Ordinarily, it would have been a relaxed affair – good food, good wine, good company. But hanging in the air was Jane's disappointment and no matter how we tried to cajole her, she couldn't see how she could even contemplate going out to Florida to do a full ironman. It seemed the adventure was over.

CHAPTER 10

September 2004

JANE

Now the Nice event was over, I felt much more relaxed. The butterflies I'd felt in my stomach on the flight over to France had long gone but now, as we settled into our seats for the return journey, all I could feel was bitter disappointment weighing down on me. Ryan had done his best to uplift me, complaining that the cutoff times for the event were far too harsh and that the bike course was too hard. He said I'd easily manage the longer times for Florida – but I just wasn't sure I wanted to put myself through it.

'You know what I think?' Mike said, as we discussed it yet again as we passed over France. I drew a breath in and waited for him to tell me. 'You should go for it. If you don't have a go this year, you'll never be this fit again. You've been training for two years.'

I rested my head back against the seat and looked out of the window where the fluffy clouds had formed a blanket beneath us. I closed my eyes and tried to imagine myself taking part in the Florida Ironman. It was just six weeks away. I knew I would be able to do the four kilometre swim but could I get fit enough to be able to complete a 180 kilometre bike ride? When Luke and I had done that distance on the 'Rome to Home' ride, it had nearly finished us off – and that was with two of us pedalling. And what about my running? Would the pain in my back and hips allow me to complete a full marathon at the end of the swim and the bike ride?

But Mike was right. I'd dreamt about this possibility for two years. If I didn't go for it this year – if I didn't even try – I would always regret it. I turned to face Mike. 'I think I should have a go and see if my health holds out.'

He smiled and thrust his fist in the air. 'Yes!' he cried. 'You know it's the right decision.' I sat back in my seat and refastened my seat belt for our descent. 'Can I tell Sara that you're definitely going?' he asked.

'I don't know,' I said. Making the decision to do it was one thing, telling the media was another. The publicity it might generate frightened me nearly as much as the challenge itself.

'I need to know because they'll have to organise everything if they're going to come out.'

I sensed there was no going back. 'Oh, okay then, tell them if you must.' As soon as Mike had told people what I was planning I began to have second thoughts. I was keeping to a hard training regime – swimming three times a week, two of those for one and a half hours at a time, cycling four to five times a week and running three times a week.

I set the turbo trainer up in the living room and watched gardening programmes as I pedalled away. By taping the remote control of the television to the bike I could channel hop to relieve the boredom of sitting crouched on the bike for three or four hours at a time.

In order to travel to Florida I needed permission from one of my doctors, for my travel insurance. I needed to be declared fit for travel, or else my insurance company would not cover me for the trip.

Mike came with me to the hospital. Dr Perrin stared at me over the small oval of his glasses, his eyebrows arched over his face, creases of concern round his eyes. 'So what are you up to now?' he asked.

'I'm thinking of going to Florida to take part in an ironman triathlon,' I said.

'Ah, yes.' His face broke into a grin. 'Remind me again what that entails.'

'A four kilometre swim, a one hundred and eighty kilometre bike ride and then you run a marathon,' I said, watching him to gauge his reaction.

'Oh, just a marathon to run,' he said. 'Are you sure you should be doing this?'

'No, not really, but I'd really like to try,' I said.

Dr Perrin looked resigned. 'I'm not entirely

happy,' he said. 'But if you must, you will be careful – that's an awfully long way to go, it's a lot to put your body through.'

'I know,' I said. 'I'm trying to make sure I'm as well prepared as possible.'

'And how much training are you doing just now?' he asked.

'About fifteen hours a week. Swimming, biking and running.'

'Well, only you know if you're fit for this. But I trust there isn't any more madness after this,' he said, looking at Mike.

'Trust me,' Mike said. 'This is the last thing we're doing.'

'What's with the we?' I asked. 'Are you taking part as well?'

'Well, emotionally,' Mike said, 'I'll be with you all the way.'

MIKE

I unclipped my black bow tie and undid the top button as soon as we got clear of the York Racecourse. We had been invited to a dinner there by the *Yorkshire Post* newspaper to celebrate their 250-year anniversary.

Unfortunately, a lovely evening had been partially blighted because Jane had been sitting next to a rather rotund female politician from East Yorkshire whose tact and diplomacy left a lot to be desired. When she wasn't earbashing a newspaper finance director she was instructing Jane as to how exactly she should be coping with cancer. Jane, to her credit, showed immense restraint, excusing herself from the table and going to the loo when most of us would have told the woman to shut up.

'What an obnoxious woman,' Jane said as we made our way to the car. 'Typical politician – up their own arse.'

It was one in the morning and there was an eerie silence as we walked past the paddock, through the turnstiles. Our route back to the car was lit by the orange glow of York's early morning street lights. Jane was clearly in some discomfort and as soon as she was seated in the passenger seat she kicked off her shoes.

'If I'd known we'd be standing for so long, I'd have worn flat shoes,' she said, bending over to rub her soles.

'Are you all right?' I asked.

'Yes, it's just the shoes.'

'We should have left a couple of hours ago.'

'We can't, it's rude.'

'It's not perfect for the ironman, though, is it? Fourteen days away,' I said.

'Oh, thanks for reminding me,' Jane said, screwing up her face.

Because I'd been the designated driver, I hadn't touched a drop of alcohol at the party, so when we finally got home my mind was racing and I couldn't get to sleep. As Jane lay next to me in bed, my mind flickered over all the things I needed to do. Nothing had been organised for Florida – no flights, accommodation or insurance. As was always the case with Jane, we'd left everything to the last minute because we could never say for sure whether she would be actually taking part in an event until a few days before. Thankfully, this time, Standard Life offered to cover expenses and New Balance promised help with insurance – so at least we could cross those off my mental list.

'Ooww, fuck!' I woke with a start and turned over to see that Jane was sitting on the edge of the bed. She tentatively stood up. 'Fuck! Fuck!' she hissed, before slumping back down.

'Are you all right?' I asked.

'Shut up!' Jane shouted. 'Shit, shit, shit.' She stood again. Reaching to her bedside table she grabbed the top and used it to manoeuvre her way to the bathroom.

'What's up?'

'I don't know,' she said.

After a couple of minutes, she returned from the bathroom and I noticed a tear roll down her cheek. In short, staccato movements, she tried to get dressed.

'Do you want a tea?' she said, as she hobbled out of the bedroom. I shook my head. By now, I was wide awake. It was seven thirty and I lay there wondering whether I should go downstairs and join her or give her some space. I waited fifteen minutes before getting up and seeing if she was okay. When I got to the kitchen, Jane was seated at the table's end, looking drained.

'I think I need to go to casualty,' she said weakly. Alarm bells started ringing. Jane is never one to be melodramatic so if she said she needed treatment, she needed treatment. I tried to remain calm.

'That bad?' I said, walking over to her and

sitting down opposite. 'What's the problem?'

'I've got an immense pain through my back, pelvis and hip. I can't walk. I'm not sure if I haven't fractured something.'

'How?' I said, my mind suddenly racing. 'Why?'

'Standing on those heels last night, it's flared up the bone pain, it's just too intense.'

I stood up. 'We'll go to casualty,' I said. 'But it'll probably be all right with rest.'

Jane's shoulders dropped. 'Step forward, Dr Michael. Let's patch you up but let's not miss going to Florida,' she said.

'That's not what I meant and you know it,' I said. 'I'll get Steven up and we'll come with you.'

She shook her head. 'Just drop me off, I'll ring you when I've finished.'

We took Jane to St James's and left her there as she'd requested. She was gone for two hours and it was twelve when she called and asked me to pick her up. She hardly spoke a word on the way home, save to tell me that nothing had shown up on the X-rays. I was reluctant to ask too much in case she accused me of only caring about Florida again. But then I figured I should risk a few questions rather than be accused of not caring at all.

'What did the doctor say?' I asked, as Jane limped through the hall into the kitchen. 'When will you be able to train again?'

She didn't answer immediately. I couldn't tell whether the frown on her face was her reaction to my question or to the pain. She reached into the cupboard for something.

'They wanted to keep me in overnight and do a

CT scan,' she said.

I was puzzled. 'What's wrong? Why have you come home then?'

'What's a scan going to show? Surprise! You've got cancer everywhere. Big deal. That won't help.'

'So what you are going to do?'

'I'll rest for two or three days and then see about running,' she said. I knew this lack of training would lay heavily on her. Although it's proven that the last three weeks of training for any event don't give the competitor any extra fitness, they do help to relieve the mental stress. When you taper off before a big event it's amazing how much you are aware of your body and how many little aches and strains you develop which are psychosomatic.

'Did you ask about the ironman?'

She shook her head. 'He didn't know. I think he thought I was mad. He did say there was little chance – but he sounded fairly clueless if you ask me.'

JANE

It was a struggle pulling on my running shorts. Each jar of my hips sent pain shuddering through my back and the large muscles either side of my spine would tighten. Trying to reach my feet to ease on my socks was even more difficult.

In the kitchen, I gently raised my foot on to the chair and tied the laces, then did the same with the other foot. Once ready, I sat for a few moments gently stretching my back, trying to stop the spasm.

'Right, I'm off,' I called to Mike, who was in the living room. 'I'm only going to the other side of the park and back.'

'Are you sure you're up to it?' he said.

'I don't know, but I might as well give it a go. I've got nothing to lose.'

I walked down the small incline towards the park, stretching my stride to test my left hip. Crossing the road, I pushed down on my right leg and set off into a very gentle jog, but as my left heel hit the ground a sharp pain shot through my pelvis. I persevered, shortening my stride to see if that would help, but when my left heel hit the ground once more, the pain remained the same.

I tried a few more strides, then walked gently again for a few minutes. Giving it another shot, I set off once again but the effect was the same. I hadn't even reached the park gates before I turned round and headed back for home. Tears of pain and frustration rolled down my face. I opened the door and Mike stood in front of me.

'I couldn't run at all. It's too sore still.'

'Let me give Dave Hancock a ring at Leeds United,' he said. 'I'm sure he'll see you. It's worth a try. You can't go on like this.'

Dave was the football team's physiotherapist. He had helped us in the past and had let us know that he was always available if we needed any help. This seemed like a time to ask for expert advice. I nodded at him. 'Yes, okay. I might as well. I'm not going to Florida like this.'

Dave agreed to see me and Mike drove me to the Leeds United training ground in Wetherby. We waited in the dining area while he finished treating the players and then he came out to greet us.

'Jane,' he said, walking over. 'Come this way.' I followed him through the corridors to the treatment room. Dave had a muscular build and he moved quickly with a purpose. He was cheerful, with a professional manner.

'Stand against the wall,' he said. I stood facing the wall while Dave looked at my posture. 'Do you always stand with your left foot like that?' he asked. I was standing with my left heel just slightly off the ground. It helped stop the pulling at my hip, which was extremely painful.

'No, but it's more comfortable than putting it flat on the ground,' I said.

His face creased, and he looked intently at my posture. He then asked me to raise my leg on one side then the other and for me to kick my leg out in front – all the time he was watching me closely. When we had finished we sat facing one another.

'There's a lot of dysfunction there which is coming from your lower back,' he said. 'Your pelvis is very stiff.'

I nodded. 'Is there anything you can suggest to help?'

His mouth closed, his hands moved, clenching and unclenching gently, while he considered his options. 'I wouldn't normally touch someone with your history with a barge pole,' he said. 'But I think if we can manipulate your back that would free up your pelvis and allow you to stretch out the tightness. You understand what might happen if I try this and your back is weak?'

'Yes, I know. I might end up going out of here on a stretcher,' I said. 'Is it worth a try though?'

'Well, I'm willing to do this but you'll have to trust me and put a lot of faith in me to allow me to treat you properly.' He looked at me, searching my face for any doubts.

I had none and I nodded firmly. 'If you're happy that's fine with me.'

'Well, I don't know about happy,' he said. 'I need you to get up on the table.'

Mike had been sitting watching all of this and he nodded his approval and reassurance. I climbed up on to the treatment table and lay flat as Dave asked, then he gathered my arms round his neck and lifted my body forward. There was a loud crack and I could feel something relax in my back at the same time. I lay on the table not daring to move. 'Right. Let's check that.' Dave watched me stand once more. My left heel met the floor with ease. The large muscle group in my back had relaxed for the first time in many weeks, and was now no longer pulling my hip joint tight and high.

'That's much better already,' he said and had me lay on my back while he worked his fingers through the tight muscles in my groin and through my thigh, stretching my leg to keep the muscle free.

The gym at the training ground had been set up by Dave and there was a swimming pool with an area for rehabilitation for the football players. I was given access to the facilities and over the next few days I returned as often as possible.

The pool was particularly useful, it was shallow enough to run through but deep enough to take the impact of the hard surface from beneath the feet. So I was able to work the muscle groups for running without stressing them.

Dave saw me a few days later and he stretched my back, once more releasing the tension that had built up. 'Have you managed to run at all yet?' he said.

'No, I've got to admit to being a bit afraid to.'

'Well, there's the training ground out there, I think you should try a gentle run. Don't push yourself and drop to a walk if you feel any tightness.'

I was a little apprehensive, but I pulled on my trainers, this time finding I was able to reach my feet with ease, but still wary of setting off any pain. Walking out to the ground I stretched the calf muscles and hamstrings very gently. Then I set off, gently at first, around the edge of the training pitch. My left heel hit the ground and there was a slight tightness but no pain. I moved round the ground. My pace was slow, my steps shorter than normal, but as my confidence increased I could stretch my stride more and more, and I slowly worked my speed up. I walked the last few yards and returned to Dave.

'How was that?' he asked.

'Fine – still just a little tight but I could feel that tightness going as I ran,' I said.

'Great. Well, if there's anything else you need just give us a shout,' he said.

'Thanks. You've done so much already. I wouldn't even be able to think about running if it weren't for you.'

'When is it you're setting off?'

'Thursday.'

'Keep doing those stretches, especially on the plane, to keep that joint moving. Do you think you're going to finish?'

'Who knows now,' I said, shrugging. 'I'll just be happy to get to the start.'

MIKE

At home that evening, after eating a hastily prepared meal of pasta, Jane, Rebecca, Steven and I sat in the kitchen to discuss whether or not we should travel to Florida. We always consulted the children on major decisions like this. It was their choice every bit as much as it was ours. If we went, they would be coming with us and if they didn't want to go – or they didn't want their mum to compete – we'd take their views on board.

Jane was still in the kit she'd been wearing when she'd been treated by Dave down at the Leeds training ground. Steven, for two minutes at least, left his Yu-Gi-Oh cards unattended to take part in this grown-up conversation, while Rebecca sat languidly in her chair, twiddling with her zip on her jumper, feigning mild disinterest as only a teenager can.

'When do we have to decide?' asked Steven.

'Tonight,' Jane said. 'It's important that you have a voice and have a say whether we go or not.'

'Are you well enough?' asked Rebecca.

'I am well enough to travel, but I don't know about competing.'

'What did Mr Perrin say?'

'Dr Perrin,' Jane corrected her. 'He wasn't there, but another oncologist said he would sign me fit to travel but that wasn't to say that I could compete. Only I could decide that.' She paused, then asked Rebecca, 'What do you think?'

'Do what you want.'

'Do you think we should go or not?'

Rebecca, her fingers hidden in the cuffs of her sleeves, still fiddled with the zip on her jumper. 'I don't know. It's up to you.'

'Steven?' Jane said.

'I'd go,' he said enthusiastically.

Rebecca laughed. 'You would say that – you just want some time off school.'

'No, I don't,' he said defensively.

'Mike?' said Jane.

'Well, I'd go on the understanding that you don't feel obliged to race. It's four days to the event. You may recover and be fit to compete. You'll kick yourself if you stay in Leeds.'

'He wants a holiday as well...' Rebecca said.

'Everything's paid for, Jane,' I said. 'There's nothing to lose.'

Jane didn't say a thing. We all sat silently, waiting for her to speak. After what seemed like for ever, she said, 'Okay, let's travel.'

Steven jumped off the stool and danced around shouting, 'Yes.' Rebecca, despite her teenage truculence, smiled. I put my arms around Jane and her upper body began to relax and slide back into me.

Four days later and by the time we arrived in Tallahassee – Florida's state capital – it was dusk. The two BBC Sarahs were arriving tomorrow, while Dave and Phil from Yorkshire Television had decided to drive from Atlanta direct to Panama City Beach, the location for the ironman. That left seven of us – myself, Jane, Mick, Becca and Steven in one people carrier while Lia and Ryan took a sporty red car.

Panama City was a massive but unattractive city and as we passed through it there were various murmurings in the car that we were glad we'd chosen to stay at Panama City Beach a few miles up the coast. But our relief was to be short-lived. Panama City Beach was a dump. The Gulf of Mexico was to our left though we had to take the map's word for it as dozens of concrete monstrosities – ostensibly hotels – blocked our view of the beach. To the right of the road were properties which were little better than wooden shacks with corrugated iron roofs – some of which had been damaged in the recent hurricanes. It was ten o'clock on a Thursday night but I'd seen more life in Settle at six o'clock on a Sunday morning. It was like a 'closed' Blackpool – without the tower, tourists or class.

'What the hell is this?' I said as Mick pulled the car into the driveway of our hotel, a three-storey-high building that wouldn't have looked out of place in a 1960s city centre council estate.

'Is this is it?' Steven said with more than a hint of disappointment.

There was a small kiosk in a separate building

in the middle of the car park and we headed there, accompanied by Ryan and Lia. A bleached blonde with a stained chequer-patterned uniform slowly removed her flip-flop feet from the counter. She slouched forward on to her elbows.

'Good day y'all,' she said in a pained southern drawl. 'I'm Cindy, who are y'all?'

'We should be booked under Tomlinson,' I said.

She looked down her list: 'Tom in son.'

'Yes.'

'From England?'

'Yes...' I said slowly, wary that communicating in words of more than one syllable might delay our check-in by hours.

Cindy made no effort to show us the rooms. She passed us our keys and turned up the TV and placed her white scarred legs on to the counter.

'I don't like it here,' Steven said.

JANE

I couldn't sleep – jet lag, the worry about my hip, the big day tomorrow. I lay in bed next to Mike, listening to the crash of waves against the shore. What if the waves are too big for me to swim in, I thought. My mind darted from one worry to another, and I kept on going over the contents of each of the bags I had packed for the different disciplines. Did I put the socks in with my cycle shoes? Three bags were already packed and laid out in transition halls. There was nothing I could do now about them but still I worried.

A noise like light pebbles being thrown against the windows stopped my brain working through the contents of the bags and I pulled the covers back from the bed and placed my feet on the floor. Easing the shutter open I could hear the full force of the sea throwing itself against the sands, the spray arcing high. The window was battered by the rain, which had been blown in under the balcony by the force of the wind. I could make out the palm trees around the pool area, they were bent with the gusts, their trunks parallel to the shoreline. The palm leaves were thrown forward and then the whole tree snapped back as the wind quietened. Then once more, it bent under the will of the winds. I closed the shutter and crept back to my bed, pulling the covers up over me. I watched the slits of light on the ceiling, willing sleep to come, hoping the storm would pass over.

I must have had some sleep because the next thing I remember is feeling for the small black alarm clock and pushing the switch to silence it. Mike slept on and I drew the covers back from me, swinging my legs round and on to the floor so as not to jar my hip.

I could see slits of light from the closed shutters but the room was dark, dawn a long way from now – it was still only 4 a.m. I sat in the small kitchen area of the room with a warm coffee and two slices of toast and chewed methodically, my throat dry with nerves, my whole self still not fully conscious. I struggled to swallow the toast but the warm milky coffee helped. I needed this fuel for the first part of the day. It was still too early to take my painkillers so I put the foil strip into my bag for later.

After eating, I started to feel more awake. I pulled on my black lycra shorts and small vest top. In the bathroom I smeared Sudocrem on to my sensitive saddle area to reduce chaffing. Over these two small clothing items I would later be pulling on my wetsuit, but for now I wanted to stay warm so I pulled on a thick jumper and some baggy combat trousers.

I closed my eyes, still heavy with sleep. Then I opened them and circled my neck to relieve the stiffness. My tense shoulders were making their way up to my ears, my nerves causing me to hold myself taut. I tried to loosen up, stretching and relaxing my neck muscles.

There was a tap at the door and I fumbled with the lock. Ryan's hair was standing up in a freshly washed shock. Small dark rings under his eyes showed his tiredness too.

'Are you ready for the off?' he asked. I nodded and retreated into the room to pick up my carrier bag. The sky was just starting to lighten and as we stood outside I could tell the wind had dropped. The day was calm.

Sara and Sarah were waiting for us and they slid the door of their car open. We all sat in silence, the early hour killing any attempts at conversation. As we drew near to the starting area we could see a steady stream of triathletes and their supporters walking towards it. The heaviness of sleep started to retreat, replaced by a tight nervous bubble of anticipation behind my breastbone.

We jumped down from the car. 'We'll see you

by your bikes in about half an hour,' Sara said.

'Yeah, that should be fine,' Ryan replied for me. I was too nervous for speech now, the dryness in my mouth locking it closed.

'I just want to see what the swim course looks like,' Ryan said and we walked alongside the hotel to the small raised dune. I looked out to the platform far out to sea, squinting to check if it really was where I was swimming to. The bubble of anticipation turned hard in my chest, my mouth too dry to swallow. The knot at the back of my throat caused a rising nausea as I started to panic. I turned and sat with my back to the sea. I didn't want to see the waves in case they were too large to swim through but I could hear the spray as they hit the beach running up the sands before pulling back to the mass of water.

Ryan returned. 'Right, let's get to transition and check out the bikes,' he said. We headed back towards the hotel. 'The water looks lovely,' Ryan said. 'It's perfect for the swim.'

Our bikes were hung on racks suspended by their saddles. I lifted mine down and Ryan pulled a long track pump from his kit bag to inflate the tyres. I lined up gel sachets and power bars to tape to the bike frame when he had finished. I pulled out two tall water bottles upending the drinks in them; water in one and an isotonic energy drink in the other. My bike was ready and I hung it back beside the others. Loaded down now with fuel for the day, it was much heavier. I walked to Ryan's bike and watched him as he went through the same routine we had just completed for my bike. I sat on the kerbside, felt the gravel through my trousers and hugged my knees to my chin.

'What time is it?' Ryan asked.

'Just coming up to six o'clock. Is it too early to get changed?'

'No, I think it's about time to get ourselves ready.'

I tugged open my bag and found the foil strip of painkillers, popping two into my hand I swallowed them down with some water. I pulled a gel sachet out and opened that, squeezing the contents into my mouth. The sweetness made me shudder as I swallowed it down. I took a long pull from my water bottle and sipped for a moment feeling the lump slowly descend into my stomach.

I pushed my feet into my wetsuit and worked the tight neoprene up my leg, rolling a large black lump up and up so that it would fit snugly. We could put off the moment no longer and followed other black-suited individuals, goggles hung round their necks, coloured hats clasped tightly in their hands.

The tight bubble of fear was growing and expanding in my chest, making it hard to breathe. My eyes narrowed in concentration at just drawing the next breath in and then out, pulling air into my lungs. I could feel my cheeks flush, the adrenalin rush tingling in my fingers and the fronts of my thighs. I trembled, shivering at the thought of the day's endeavours as I looked out to sea following the markers once more.

I sat down on the sandy beach hugging myself tightly, placing my forehead on my knees, and pushed out the noise and fervour of the others around me. I said a silent prayer, thanking God for bringing me to this place, asking for courage to meet the endeavours before me and finally requesting a safe day, whatever the outcome, whether I finished or had to admit defeat.

'Good luck,' I said to Ryan.

'You too. Have a safe one.'

'You too.'

The hooter sounded and we walked with 2000 other triathletes into the water. The thrashing of arms and legs turned the water into one giant wave surging out to sea. I spread my arms wide to create a space around me, pushing a large man to my right as I started swimming.

Keeping Ryan's cap in view I swam my long slow freestyle. Three strokes and then a breath, three strokes and then I looked and spotted Ryan's cap to the left. Another three strokes, another breath. The bubbles of all the swimmers in front of me seemed to pull me along, making my body feel light in the water. I rode the wave of the swimmers past buoy after buoy, cutting through the water with ease until at last I could see the turn and we were heading back to shore. I tagged on to a group of swimmers and eased back to the shore. Feeling sand under my feet, I waded out on to the beach and headed back into the water for the second lap.

'Come on, Jane. You're doing really well. Fantastic swimming.' It was Mike.

I could see a group of strong swimmers ahead. I headed for the rear of that group and pulled myself through the water. Reaching the turn far out at sea I started to tire. My arms felt heavier, my breathing harsher. I inhaled seawater and felt it flowing up and down my airways as I forced air past it into my lungs.

At last, I felt sand once more under my feet and I waded out of the water. Coughing to try to clear the water from my lungs, I could hear Mike shouting and see Steven bouncing beside him.

'Well done, Jane!'

'What time was that?' I asked him as I passed.

He ran through the other spectators keeping up with me. 'One hour thirty-six,' he yelled. 'Absolutely awesome.'

I turned myself in the showers provided for the swimmers, trying to wash the salty water from myself. Groups of volunteers helped remove wet suits, so I sat and waited for them to come to me so they could tug the suit down and over my legs. When it was my turn, I clutched my left thigh to stop any jarring of my hip, grabbed the wet suit from the outstretched arm and yelled 'thank you' before heading for the hall to pick up my bike bag.

My head was light, my eyes unfocused, my legs wobbled beneath me. The oxygenated blood from my upper torso and arms flooded into the rest of my body. I shook my head to gather myself.

Pulling on my cycling shorts and a cycle top I sat and tugged on socks – my left sock wouldn't sit right and at the third attempt I finally managed to get the heel of the sock into the correct place. I unscrewed the top of the flat bottle of Coke and sipped. I wanted to dilute the salty water in my stomach so I could take on the carbohydrates from the gels and bars later. I pushed my feet into shoes and smeared sun cream on to my arms and legs and the back of my neck, recalling my experience at the Nice triathlon. I swallowed the contents of a caffeinated gel sachet, hoping the sugar rush would clear the blurring in my vision. Helmet on, I moved out to the transition area where I wheeled my bike through to the start line and mounted it and set off with Ryan in my wake.

My legs felt sluggish, my stomach churned with the brine of the sea gurgling through my innards. I tried to keep low on the bike, streamlined to reduce my speed, and then sat more upright to relieve the discomfort in my belly.

An hour into the ride and I'd covered fifteen miles which was my target. But I felt bad. 'I don't feel too good,' I shouted at Ryan's back.

'It's too early to start moaning,' he called and dropped back so that he was riding alongside me for just a moment. My legs were turning but my heart wasn't in it. 'Come on!' yelled Ryan. 'Get down on your tri bars. You drop a minute a mile when you're down on those.'

I looked at him and he glared back at me, daring me to argue. Clenching my jaw I lowered my body and stretched my arms long on to the bars, circling my legs smooth and fast.

'That's it,' he said. 'We'll stop at the next aid station. See how you feel then.'

I nodded and watched as he slid smoothly past me with just a few turns of his legs. We reached the first aid station half an hour later.

'Do you need to stop?' Ryan asked and I shook my head, unscrewing the lid from my bottle. I was feeling slightly better now that my body was accustomed to the cycling. I placed the lid in my back pocket and stretched out to reach for a bottle of Gatorade to replenish my drink. The fluid glugged as it flowed into the bottle and I screwed the cap back on. I kept moving, the nerves and fears of the hours before me receding as the miles passed under my wheels.

At the next aid station fifteen miles on, we both stopped and I climbed off my bike. With the same rolling gait as my fellow competitors, my legs weaving underneath me, I walked to the portaloo and waited.

Afterwards, having relieved some of the pressure from my belly, I grabbed the bike by its main stem and steered it out to the roadside. Once more lifting my leg over the crossbar, I set off. A tall man, his dark baseball cap covering white blond hair, held out a bottle of water. I reached for it and took some sips before throwing it to the ground near the refuse sacks.

'You're awesome man,' he shouted. 'You're on your way back home now.'

His fervour brought a smile to my face. 'Thank you,' I yelled at him and moved off.

'You took your time,' Ryan said as we reached the halfway point. I screwed my nose up at him. I watched him circling his legs faster than mine and concentrating, making them move faster then faster still. We came to a small wooded area. The shade was a welcome relief – the temperature no lower but it felt good to be out of the incessant glare of the sun, which was now high up in the sky.

'Look at that,' shouted Ryan, pointing over to the side of the road. There was a sign pushed into the turf. 'GO, JANE TOMLINSON, GO!' and in smaller letters 'GOOD LUCK, GIRL'. I laughed out loud to see support so many miles from home.

After eighty miles, there was still two hours' cycling to go and my legs were tiring, my back was in knots. The road surface was poor, made up of concrete sections and with each section, pain would judder through my shoulders, elbows and hands down to my hips, knees and feet. Bump bump bump – I stared down at the straight road. At each thud of the tyre, dark spots of sweat dropped from my body and I could see them explode into a tiny universe as they hit the dusty tarmac. I tried to sit lightly on the bike but my legs were too tired.

I was eating energy bars and taking in gel sachets every thirty minutes as well as sipping at water and energy drinks steadily throughout the day. I knew I needed to stop my body sugar from dropping.

'How are you doing?' Ryan called as we neared the only hill on the course. I changed to a small gear to allow my legs to ease round and round and climb the slight gradient.

'I'm feeling very sick,' I said. 'Does it matter if I can't eat anything?' I knew what his answer would be but I also knew I would throw up if I forced anything else down.

A small frown crossed his face before he answered. 'No,' he lied. 'That's fine, just keep drinking, even if you do feel ill.'

From the look on his face, I could tell he was concerned so I slipped my hand down to my bottle and tipped water into my mouth. I swirled it around and spat it into the kerbside, then took a long sip and swallowed it down. It sat on my stomach and my belly gurgled in protest.

After my initial dismay and low morale at the beginning of the ride, I passed each aid station with growing elation. I could do this. We passed another marker and the finish was just under fifteen miles away. I knew that I would get there and even my nausea couldn't drive away the smile that was starting to creep up my face.

As we neared the transition area, the loneliness of the long ride was relieved by the crowds that lined the streets, clapping and cheering as we passed. A dark van was stopped in a lay-by. The door opened and Mike and Steven erupted from its depths.

'Come on, Jane! Fantastic effort!' Mike cried.

'Go, Mum, go!' cheered Steven. The smile spread further across my face. The tiredness in my body momentarily forgotten, my legs spun strongly once more.

In a matter of seconds, I could see the arch that marked the end of the bike section, and I came to a halt. Forcing my leg over the crossbar, I dismounted and wheeled my bike forward. My legs moved woodenly, my hips unused to anything but the smooth rotation of the pedals. My feet thumped heavily against the ground as I walked to the transition area. The bike was taken from me by an official, and I gave it up gratefully. I looked at my watch, but my mind was too tired to work out how long I'd been on the bike. I could see it was just past four o'clock so that would give me just under eight hours to run the marathon. For the first time that day I began to believe that I might see the finish line.

Sitting in the changing area of the transition hall I pulled off my cycling top, forcing myself to stand and tug at my cycling shorts. Delving in my plastic bag, I pulled out my running cap and water bottle. I sat back down on the chair, frozen against it, unable to make my body move. Sitting looking idly around me, I stared at other women readying themselves for the run. A helper came over and pulled me back to the present.

'Do you need anything?' she asked, gathering my bag for me. I shook my head, rousing myself, and bent to tie the laces of my trainers. I picked up my treat for the day – a small packet of savoury cheese crackers – then with an enormous effort I pushed myself upright and made my way out to the start of the run.

'Jane! How are you?' Mike asked. He was standing at the run exit. I nodded at him.

'Fine,' I called. I was too weary and dazed to seek any other vocabulary to reassure him.

'You can do it now,' he called, as I forced myself onwards, out on to the run course. I started running slowly, but didn't get very far before stomach cramps forced me to walk. Ryan eased alongside me.

'Try eating something,' he said. I took a small cracker from the packet I was clutching and pushed it into my mouth. Chewing it slowly, I was surprised to find that after the sweet drinks and energy bars, the savoury crumbly cracker was a pleasant change. I washed it down with water and started running again, my legs feeling stronger as I moved further onwards, the familiar running sensation returning to them after the long cycle ride. It was a slow run, but I forced myself steadily onwards, one foot in front of the other, heading towards the first mile marker.

MIKE

Like a test-match slip-fielder waiting for a catch from every ball, I found myself tensing up each time a runner came into view – only to relax again when I realised it wasn't Jane. It was a two lap there-and-back course so the spot where we'd decided to pitch up on the side of the road became the 4, 9, 17 and 22 mile points of the run. We stood on a corner near a feed station so that we could have two long uninterrupted views of the course and it seemed a perfect place to spot Jane.

As I stood at the side of the course looking out for her, Steven sat on the ground playing with his Game Boy, while Rebecca, her back propped against the wall, legs out in front of her, chatted to Mick. The two Sarahs stood with me, keeping a watching brief.

'What time is it, Mick?' I asked.

'Five past seven.'

When Jane had first come past us at the four-mile mark, dusk was just beginning to close in but now it was completely dark. I computed some timings in my head. With five hours left, and at the speed she'd set off at, I figured she had more than enough time to complete the run – it was just a question of whether her fragile body would allow her to finish. Of course, she'd done a marathon before – the London 2004 – when she was injured and poorly but this was different as she'd already been competing for nine hours. After she had started her swim in the morning we'd had a straw poll as to whether she'd finish and out of the fourteen of us, only Phil Iveson from Yorkshire Television was positive.

'I've seen her worse than this at Rome before she set off,' he said. 'No one gave her a chance there and she did it.'

Suddenly, from round the bend, Jane came into view, looking absolutely knackered. She was shuffling rather than running, her head down looking at the ground.

'Come on, Jane,' I shouted, then turned to Steven, 'Steven! It's Mum.'

He jumped up and joined me at the side of the road, as did Rebecca and Mick. Ryan pulled away from Jane and sprinted ahead to me quickly.

'How is she?' I asked.

'Her hip's not good, sir,' he said.

'Will she finish?' I asked and he held out his hand horizontally, tipping it from side to side as if to say 50-50 chance.

'Shit,' I muttered. Jane approached slowly. She was struggling, there could be no doubt about it. Her shoulders were drooped, her head lolloping about, she didn't even look up when I yelled.

'Come on, Jane,' I shouted and ran to her side, joining her for fifty yards and yelling encourage-ment. Still, she said nothing, just ground out yard after yard before turning a corner and disappearing. I stood there watching the empty space, wondering if she'd make it back on the return lap.

'I'm hungry!' Steven interrupted my thoughts.

'Shall we get off, grab some food then get to transition?' I said to him, figuring it would take Jane at least forty-five minutes at her present pace to get to the point where she would have to turn round and return on the final lap.

'Did she look all right to you?' I said to no one in particular as we piled into the people carrier. 'She looked knackered to me. Did you see how she was running? Do you think she's okay? Did you hear her say anything? I didn't hear her say anything...'

'Calm down, Dad...' Steven said. 'I keep telling you not to worry. Mum's all right.'

Rebecca chortled at her little brother's confidence. 'Well said, Steven. Give me five.'

We dropped Sarah and Rebecca off at the finish line and headed for Burger King. During mid-afternoon at the transition area, which was located behind the finishing line, we'd already seen some of the fastest competitors finish the contest – and what a distressing sight that was. These were athletic young men who in the heat of the late Florida sun had pushed their bodies past their physical limit in the hope of clipping seconds from their personal bests.

We saw them approaching the finishing line in their dozens, inebriated with exhaustion and collapsing unconscious to the floor – their poor bodies unable to move an inch further. Medical staff would rush over, haul them on to one of the many stretchers that lay waiting at the finishing line before attaching saline drips to their arms while they tried to bring them round. The two Sarahs, who had waited at the finishing line to film those first past the post, soon decided to turn the cameras off. This wasn't suitable viewing for a documentary about Jane. Meanwhile, I had shepherded Steven out of sight – we'd look out for his mum further down the course.

JANE

The first half of the marathon had not been so bad. The first mile had been the hardest, as I struggled to fall into a running action after so long in the saddle. After that, I had been able to maintain a steady pace for most of the thirteen miles, stopping regularly at drinks stations to revive myself with tepid chicken soup and sweet energy drinks.

The first thirteen miles had taken me about 2 hours and 40 minutes, but this last half was slow and hard. I was walking more than running. When I did manage to run, it was slow and I was unable to keep up the action for any length of time.

My eyes were tired and kept closing. Each time I opened them, my head would snap back and I'd see Ryan several yards ahead of me, urging me forward. I used the sight of the back of his shirt to pull me onwards, attaching a mental rope to it to tug me towards him.

'Right Jane,' he turned and said as we fell into

yet another slow walk. 'When we get to the next lamppost we'll start running.' His tone was reasonable but firm, not to be argued with.

'Which one?' I asked, squinting ahead in the gloom of the gathering night.

'That one, just ahead,' he said, pointing. I could see it now and nodded, but carried on walking, the water bottle in my hand dropping to my side, thumping against my thigh. I forced my feet to move onwards to the circle of light in the distance. We arrived at the lamppost and I pushed against the ache in the midpoint of my thighs and forced my legs into a running action. Except they wouldn't obey the command my mind was sending, they were stubbornly resisting my will. I tried again and managed to gain enough momentum to run a few strides before my legs rebelled once more and I had to drop back to a slow halting excruciating walk.

'I think I'd like to go home now,' I mumbled through my dry mouth. Ryan turned his face to me but I was unable to read the expression on his still features. He considered my words for a long moment.

'I'm going to run on ahead to the next drink station and wait for you there,' he said. I didn't have the energy to protest and watched with envy as he ran with ease on ahead of me, making a mockery of my sorry efforts.

'Come on, Jane,' I growled, low and fierce, as my legs protested under me. Gritting my teeth and ignoring the pain I edged closer until I drew alongside him. He passed me a cup of thin chicken broth and I sipped from it.

'Come on, keep it up for a little longer,' he said. The small mental victory of catching him up gave me a boost to carry on a little further, to the next lamppost and then the next. Up to the sign at the corner, round the bend. My goal of completing the ironman was now reduced to tiny steps met, forcing me slowly onwards to the finish.

'Sorry about leaving you back there,' Ryan said. 'I didn't know what to say to you to keep you going. I figured you wouldn't give in while you were chasing me.'

'I guessed what you were doing,' I said. 'That doesn't stop me thinking you're a bastard, though, for doing it.' I spoke slowly; I could hear my voice as though it were someone else's. My words were spoken slowly, syllable by syllable, like some drunk trying to pretend they were sober.

'My legs are cold,' Ryan said as we moved onwards.

'Ha!' I crowed. 'You thought I was wasting time pulling on my running tights. Who's sorry now?'

We came to the next drinks station and I stood for a moment to sip at some cool water. I was going to allow myself to walk for five minutes then it was time to run once more.

'Right, run again,' Ryan commanded. This time my legs obeyed and we set off at a slow jog that seemed to me to be slower than my walking pace. Passing the street lights, their halos glared in my eyes and I pulled the peak of my running cap lower over my face. We had covered a lot of ground on this last run effort and I was just about to drop to a walk once more when we rounded a corner and I saw Lia.

'Go, Jane, go!' she called, running alongside me with her small camera held in front of her, catching my feeble attempts at a marathon on film. 'Mike's just around the corner.'

'Oh, great,' I said to Ryan. 'I'll have to carry on running now. I'm buggered if I'm going to let him see me walking after I've run so far.' We ran onwards and were greeted by Mike.

Steven stood up from the bank he had been resting on. 'Go on, Mum. Go on,' he yelled. I turned as I past him and waved.

'You're unbelievable,' Mike was shouting. 'It's absolutely amazing. You're nearly there. Not far now. I'll see you at the finish.' I smiled at him, forcing my mouth from the grimace of pain to a tired grin. We rounded the corner and I fell to a walk.

'I can't run any more,' I whined at Ryan. 'You don't need to,' Ryan said. 'You can walk to the finish from here. You are running through the finishing line though.'

'Of course,' I said. We walked on.

'I've always wanted to run a marathon with a glow stick,' Ryan said. We'd been given the loops of plastic that glowed in the dark. They allowed late competitors to be visible to the referees and volunteers out on the course. They were similar to the one Steven had carried when it was bonfire night.

'Don't tell me you've never been slow enough to have the privilege before.'

Another hour passed as we headed towards the finish. I was confident that even at this pace I was going to complete the course.

'Right, Jane, the finish is round the corner. Run,' Ryan said. We could hear the PA system in the distance and see the glow of the lights at the finish. I picked my feet up for the last time, my legs obeying this final command of the day. We moved slowly towards the finish. Me, at a slow limping run, Ryan moving easily alongside me. At last I could see the barriers of the finishing chute. I could see the arch of the finish area.

'Let's hear it for Jane Tomlinson,' the man called to the small crowd gathered around the finish. 'What a tremendous effort.'

I ran onwards beside Ryan. He caught my hand and we passed through the finishing tape together with our arms aloft. Ironmen together. Two years of dreaming and training. Two years of chemo and radiotherapy. Two more years of living with my family. There were friends and family at the other side of the tape. Mike, Steven, Rebecca, Mick. None of them had believed I would finish. I was scarcely able to take in the fact that I had. I was an ironman.

I stood with Ryan's arm around my shoulder, my arm around his waist, holding the medal up from around my neck for the official finisher's photograph. 'I've finished a few ironman triathlons, but this has been the best ironman experience of any of them,' said Ryan to someone at his side. 'Finishing with Jane will be unforgettable.'

Steven, Mike and Rebecca were at my side, Steven holding Mike's hand. 'I guess we'll have to do what Mum wants to do tomorrow now, won't we, Dad?'

'No,' I said, 'we can do whatever you want to do.'

A volunteer came up to me, looking concerned. 'Do you want the medical tent or some pizza?' he asked. We walked towards the smell of the pizzas.

CHAPTER 11

February 2005

JANE

The room was silent as a list of things I had achieved over the last few years ran up a large screen like credits at the end of a TV programme. The short film finished, the lights were flicked on and I turned to face the audience.

I had been asked to speak to the England rugby team in the week before they were to play France in the Six Nations Championship. They had invited me here to chat about what motivated me and how I prepared mentally for the challenges I set myself.

I stood, shaking with nerves, trying not to catch anyone's eye for fear of my mouth seizing up and stopping me talking. I gripped the small sheets of papers containing the notes I'd made but noticed the papers fluttering in my fingers. The team remained quiet but I couldn't help but be daunted by their physical size and immense reputation.

'I expect you're wondering what relevance I have

to any of you,' I began. 'What can I, a middle-aged woman, have to talk to you about when you're elite athletes? I'm not even an athlete. What would I know about the mental preparation and motivation you might require? Standing in front of you all I feel frightened, intimidated. I'm not sure why I'm here but then I remember. I've had much more frightening experiences. Much more difficult times.

'Today will be over soon but on Thursday I've got to decide which one of three chemotherapy regimes I should choose in the hope of gaining some control of the disease that is slowly killing me. The awful thing is that none of the treatments are right for me. I have to make the best choice of the three, then I have to believe that I have made the correct decision and move on without regrets.'

I talked about my experience of the ironman, pushing my body to the limits almost without fear, to see how far it would lead me. I talked of undergoing chemo, choosing a harsh regime, and putting my body on the line to try to make sure I could achieve the goal of 'Rome to Home'.

My gamble had paid off – not only with the long bike ride but also the long distance triathlon afterwards. Things my body shouldn't be capable of I'd had to overcome – pushing limits to try to meet my goals. The rugby players seemed moved by some of the things I'd endured. I hope I motivated them too.

The next day I began chemotherapy. The regime sounded easy. Taking tablets twice a day isn't too bad but at the end of the second week I felt weak and shaky. Diarrhoea purged me and I started to pass blood as wave after wave of cramping pains twisted through my belly.

The muscles in my thighs knotted with spasms as the cramps coiled through me, leaving me curled into a foetal position covered with a blanket on the settee.

'You don't look very well,' Mike said when he arrived home one day after work. I turned my head to look at him, too tired to sit up.

'I don't feel too good,' I said. Not only was my belly hurting, my fingers were sore and my mouth was a raw mass of blisters to the very back of my throat, making it hard to swallow without excruciating pain. 'I've got a hospital appointment tomorrow.'

'Do you think you'll be okay for Saturday?' he asked. I nodded. 'Phew. Steven would have been disappointed if we had missed the England match.'

'I know. He's very excited about it.'

'Has it fired you up at all seeing the England team?' he asked.

I shrugged my shoulders. Seeing the preparations for the match and meeting the players had certainly been an experience and I had been honoured to give out the shirts for the game and to be presented with one of my own. But at that moment I couldn't get excited about anything.

At lunch with the England stars, conversation had moved to my plans for future events. We'd mentioned our latest dream – cycling across America – and Mike had now become determined to see it through.

'Don't you fancy it?' he asked, his eyes shining, a smile spread across his face. I couldn't believe he was discussing such an extreme adventure when I could hardly even walk.

'The idea's exciting,' I said. 'But I don't think I could face being in the spotlight for that amount of time.'

'You wouldn't have to be; we could make sure it was a real road trip. Go on, you know you'd enjoy it. Think what an experience it would be.'

'Seeing the England team makes me think I might want to do something, but I'm not sure, I think I've had enough of doing events. It's too demanding. I just want my life back and to enjoy the family.'

Mike shook his head. 'You'll get bored with that in a few months. You know you'll say yes. You would get to cycle across America and, if you wanted to, we'd raise a load of money for charity.'

'Yeah, I know,' I said.

'There. I knew you wanted to.'

'I haven't said yes yet.'

'I know but at least you're thinking about it.'

MIKE

Jane had worked hard to retain some fitness while on chemo. She'd insisted that this round of treatment had not been 'too bad' but one unexpected side effect had been that her hands and feet had blistered, which meant that she was unable to run.

We'd just spent four glorious days completing the Cheshire cycle way with Steven but, even so,

Jane was longing for the chemo to finish so she could get back out to train properly. She was like a caged bear and couldn't wait to get back to the Rothwell Harriers running club and begin reducing her times. Three days after her chemo finished she was back into her trainers.

I dropped her off at the club early that evening with instructions to collect her after the session. 'Don't be late,' she said and made her way to meet the rest of the group.

As I returned an hour later to collect her the trees of Springhead Park were resplendent with different shades of green. Drawing off the roundabout by Oulton Hall, the path was lined with runners making their way back to the sports centre. Slowing the car down, I scanned for Jane before spotting her running easily and chatting with some fellow athletes. My body relaxed unwittingly. I always tensed when Jane was out, perhaps subconsciously aware of the fine line she trod between staying fit and fracturing her weakened bones. My grip loosened on the steering wheel and I resumed concentration on the traffic.

Coming off another roundabout, I was distracted by the group of runners I'd just passed looking down at the ground. To my horror I saw Jane sitting on the pavement. Her face was etched with pain. My heart sank and I reversed to rejoin them. Malcolm, a genial older runner, stood over her, his hand resting on her shoulder, while Carol, another athlete, bent down beside her. I parked up next to Jane.

'She's hurt her ankle, Mike,' Malcolm said. Jane was nursing her leg, tears streaming.

'How bad is it, Jane?' I asked.

'It's okay. I'm just really mad with myself.'

I opened the passenger door and then bent down to help her. 'Is it broken?'

'I don't think so.'

With Malcolm taking one arm and me the other, we positioned her in the car and within seconds we were heading home. There were a multitude of questions I wanted to ask but I hid my curiosity. We called at home so the kids could see Mum was fine before I dropped her off at casualty.

'Is it the cancer?' I asked Jane.

'No, I'd just finished running when I went to cross the main road and slipped on the kerb. Don't make one of your crass comments. I'm cross enough for the both of us.'

'Too busy talking were you?'

'Yes. I'm furious. Five months of chemo and now this.'

'Is it broken?'

'I've already told you I don't think so. I've never broken a bone so I don't know but it's not particularly painful, certainly nothing like the pain I get from the cancer.'

Jane was home a couple of hours later, her leg in a plaster cast and we sat contemplating the implications of her broken ankle. Our family holiday was due to start in two weeks. We had planned to be cycling in the Loire. Also, Jane was due to fly for the first day of the holiday to Barcelona to give a talk to an international health conference. I looked at her.

'How could you be so stupid?'

She glared at me. 'Not a word, Mike. It's my

fault, my leg, my health. So butt out.'

JANE

My legs had lost the strength from the last few
years of running. My left ankle was stiff and I
tired easily. I had reduced my running while
having chemo because my feet blistered so badly.
After months of being unable to do anything
much physically, it was depressing having to start
again from scratch. Rebecca came out with me
for the first few runs.

'Come on, Mum,' she said on the first time we
ran. 'You're running well.'

Just at that moment my ankle started to stiffen
and I dropped to a walk. We had only run a few
hundred yards and my legs were already tired.
'We'll just walk till the next lamppost then,'
Rebecca said and so we did, resuming our slow
pace when we passed the post.

'This is hard work,' I moaned, stumbling behind
Becca feeling much older than my forty-one years.
I managed to run for another couple more minutes before my ankle tightened anew and we were
forced to walk again for a little while. It took us
over ten minutes to cover three-quarters of a mile.
I stood at the end of the road, feeling dejected. I
stretched my calf muscles and my hamstrings,
taking a few moments to regain my breath before
we turned and made our way homewards.

'It's horrible, I feel like I'm barely moving,' I
said when I eventually caught up with Rebecca at
the top of the very slight incline.

'Don't worry, it'll get easier, you'll see,' she said. And she was right. It did.

By the end of September my legs were just about strong enough to carry me thirteen miles. I knew I still had a long way to go to be fit enough for the New York Marathon at the beginning of November but the more I ran, the stronger I felt. My average time per mile slowly fell until eventually I could run about eight and a half minutes for at least the first mile. Some days were more frustrating than others. Often, I felt like I was running through treacle, my breath was wheezing and my legs heavy.

As October arrived and the days began to shorten, I stuck to training on familiar roads at night. The fog would catch at the back of my throat making the hills steeper and longer and I'd struggle to keep my head pointing upwards, willing my legs to keep moving.

A fortnight before we were due to fly out to America for the marathon, I was dreading another week of long slow painful running sessions. I looked at the hill near our home that I planned to use to try to strengthen my legs. For some reason, it seemed especially steep, the railings at the top looked further than on other days and a strong wind tried to force me down as I dropped my head and drove myself to continue. Using my arms, I slowly made my way to the top, turning round and loping to the bottom before setting off to climb it once more.

I had been dreading this particular training session, knowing how hard it would be and how much it would hurt, but it was a necessary evil. Now I was here, it was okay. The weeks of training had finally paid off as my legs moved strongly, steadily up the hill just one more time.

MIKE

My feet had swollen so much from the flight to New York that my trainers barely fastened. I tugged at the laces, undoing them then doing them up again for about the eleventh time as Jane stood next to me going through some basic stretches. The public address system was belting out a motivational tune I didn't recognise. I tied the last bow and stood up again and shook my head.

'Should you be running?' Jane asked. I was touched by her concern but also felt slightly insulted. I'd been training hard for this. Only recently, I'd run twenty miles in 3 hours 10 minutes – a remarkable time for me – but that was on a dark wet evening after work in Leeds. Today, as we limbered up at the start line on Staten Island our clothes were already slightly damp. The temperature was in the mid-seventies and humidity was at an unbearable 97 per cent.

'I'll manage,' I said but my stomach was knotting with nerves.

The early morning mist shrouding the island was beginning to lift and the colossal Verrazano-Narrows Bridge, the world's longest suspension bridge when it opened in 1964, was being seen in its glory for the first time that day. Within moments of the 'Star Spangled Banner' ending, the race began and we were shuffling slowly on to the bridge, the lower deck bouncing from the rhythmic steps of thousands of runners' feet hitting it. I was struggling before we'd even made a mile and Jane was already beginning to pull ahead. As I reached mile 6 there was no sign of her, and I was left alone to enjoy the cacophony of music – rock, hip hop, jazz – blaring out from the houses on either side of the street. They were big terraced houses with colourful doors and decorations, with steps which were packed with people shouting encouragement. There was barely an empty space. At mile 8, my feet were continuing to swell and conscious not to take on too much fluid, I rationed myself despite the humidity.

At mile 12 I took some painkillers from the medical stand and my number was marked. The squiggly black mark would ensure that no other medical control would give me painkillers during the race. Within a mile my self-discipline had vanished completely and I drank a pint Gatorade without it touching the sides.

Queens was as silent as Brooklyn was noisy. We ran through the Jewish quarter where people lined the streets in their religious dress, standing impassively, offering no encouragement. Manhattan's skyline had appeared occasionally in the distance throughout the first fifteen miles before Queensboro Bridge, a tantalising promise of the end. I'd completed the first half in 2 hours 15 which was only five minutes outside where I wanted to be. Bearing in mind it was hillier and harder on the feet than London, I was happy with that time. As I reached midpoint of Queensboro Bridge over the top of Roosevelt Island, I was idly strolling, chewing the fat with someone from Montana, when I heard Jane.

'Are you all right?' she said. By the time I'd recovered from the surprise of seeing her, she was past me and it took an effort I didn't think I had to catch her.

'How about you?' I panted.

'I'm not the one walking,' she said.

'You sarky cow.'

'Well, you could put some effort in.'

Infuriated, I kept up with her, promising to myself to whip her arse as soon as we got on to First Avenue. Dropping off the bridge and on to Manhattan the noise of the crowds was deafening, it hit you as though you were running into a wall of sound. It couldn't help but to provide an immediate lift. I was going well until the last mile when I noticed a man with a Yorkshire Cancer Research T-shirt limping so badly that, deciding to play the good Samaritan, I walked with him, encouraging him to keep going. That was until the last 100 yards when Lazarus left me for dead in a sprint finish – bastard.

Jane finished ten minutes ahead of me and once again I couldn't help but marvel at her efforts. After the race, we met up with the kids and also Ryan, who had joined us over here to help us with preparations for Jane's Ride Across America.

That evening, we went out for a meal – Ryan had been told about a great Chinese place by someone at the hotel. Rebecca, who was stalking around some glass cabinets in the restaurant, shouted over to us. 'Look at these!' she said. 'There are chopsticks signed by Bill Clinton, Tom Cruise, there's everyone.'

Jane and I looked at each other and went over to the glass cabinet where a whole array of chopsticks signed by a host of A-list celebrities was displayed.

'How much is this going to cost?' I whispered. I was about to suggest we leave when a waiter took us to our table. In jeans and T-shirt I felt woefully underdressed and I had a sensation of a hundred pairs of eyes looking down at the Hillbillies from across the Atlantic. We sat down self-consciously and picked up the menus. As I read down the list, I was mentally calculating just how much cash we had on us and how much we'd spent on the credit cards.

'I'll have crispy duck,' Rebecca said.

'No, you won't,' said Jane firmly, nodding towards the menu where crispy duck was listed at the price of $40.

'Wow,' said Rebecca, 'I'm not that hungry.'

The meal was sumptuous and we were treated kindly by the waiters, who pointed out that there would be sufficient food in one order for Rebecca and Steven to share. Jane looked at me. 'If I manage to finish the Ride Across America next year, this is where we'll come to celebrate.'

JANE

I thought the pain in my back and hips would

lessen after I had stopped the longer runs in the marathon training schedule. But it had persisted and I had asked for an appointment to see my consultant.

'So how are you?' Dr Perrin asked.

'Not too good actually,' I replied. 'I asked the nurses to change my appointment and bring it forward because I'm getting more and more pain and I'm so tired that I'm not coping very well with it.'

'Your tumour markers are within normal limits but that's not a good guide for you. Looking at the trend they seem to have been drifting upwards for the last month or so,' Dr Perrin said.

'I just feel like my disease is getting on top of me.'

'We'll get some scans done and I'll see you with the results before Christmas.'

He scribbled on to the appointments sheet and passed it to me. His script was more careful as he wrote out the request cards for the scans, one for my back and the other for my chest and abdomen.

My appointments came through promptly. I was glad; the pain had worsened. I had spoken to a nurse at a local hospice about pain control and she had given me some practical information about the morphine dosage that would help. It meant that I could control the pain better over the course of the day and sleep more easily.

Each day was a long slow process. I awoke earlier and earlier as it took me longer and longer to gain control of the pain, enough to make me more mobile. Sitting on the edge of my bed one morning, I tried to reach the sock I had dropped to the floor. My back was stiff, my left hip sore. I rocked my back forward but I still couldn't bend to pick it up. I curled the toes of my right foot up and managed to grasp the sock; bending my leg brought it into reach of my hands. I bent my left leg but my hip was too stiff for my foot to be brought to my hands. I got up from my bed and sank down slowly to the floor so that I might finish dressing myself.

'Why don't you stay at home?' Mike asked.

'I'll be all right in an hour,' I said. 'I'm just a bit stiff but I'll be fine.'

'You can barely move.'

'Oh, shut up,' I retorted, frustration and pain made my voice louder, my tone angrier than I had meant. I lifted my vest top over my head and struggled to manoeuvre my arms through the holes. I sat on the bed waiting for the spasm in my side to subside. I walked stiffly downstairs and into the kitchen.

'You're right, I'll give work a ring at nine o'clock and tell them I'm too ill to come in today. A day's rest might do me some good.'

'Well, take it easy and make sure you do rest,' Mike said. Steven shouted goodbye as they both headed for the door.

'Aren't you forgetting something, daft pants?' I called after Steven.

'What?' he asked, raising his arms and at the same instant realising that he wasn't carrying his school bag. He turned and grinned at me as he shut the door.

I was nervous about the results. It was the week before Christmas, and I had kept myself busy with the preparations for the festive season.

'Jane, do you want to come through?' Dr Perrin called and stood waiting as I pulled my bags up. 'Is Mike with you?' he glanced around and Mike stood, having shoved his book in his pocket.

We walked into the clinic, a large square room with an examination couch in one corner. Dr Perrin held the door as we walked through and shook our hands. 'Take a seat.' I hobbled for one of the two seats at the opposite side of the desk to Dr Perrin.

He sat with my notes open and the computer screen white with my latest scan reports. 'The MRI of your back shows a significant deterioration of your disease,' Dr Perrin said. 'But it's your CT scan that's more worrying. There's one larger area of tumour in your liver and a smaller one. Looking at your liver function test and all your other results it doesn't seem to be affecting the liver function so you won't have noticed any symptoms.' Mike's face was unmoving.

'That doesn't sound like good news,' I said. 'Can you explain the significance of the results? Are there any treatment options?'

I had been trying to keep myself from being emotional. This was very bad news and I wanted to be able to hold myself together to discuss the next step. 'I'm sorry,' I said as my shoulders heaved and a sob dripped from my mouth, tears flowing down my cheeks. I brushed them away but others followed. 'I was trying to be brave. I didn't think it would be good news but I don't

400

want to cry.'

Dr Perrin stood and walked across the room to pick up a small box of tissues. I grabbed a couple and wiped the tears from my face. Balling the soggy tissue in my palm, I felt calmer and sat looking at the doctor.

'Taking into account the scan results and your blood tests, we would normally say to someone whose disease was this far advanced that they were looking at around one year from this diagnosis.' I nodded. I felt that the inevitable was happening. My disease was marching on through my body. My uncertain future looked a lot shakier.

'What about treatment options?'

'There are a couple of options but you've responded well to Herceptin in the past and I think we could start with that and give it weekly with chemotherapy as well. You should tolerate Taxol quite well and giving Herceptin weekly might reduce the chance of the cardiac problem recurring.' I nodded my agreement and Mike looked a little bit less tense now that treatment was being proposed.

'We'll need to get some cardiac function tests done quite promptly but I think we should go ahead and start treatment while you are waiting for your scan appointment to come through.'

Mike sat upright in his chair. 'Jane was thinking about cycling across the USA next year. What do you think her chances of getting there are?'

'If it was anyone else I would say none. As it's you I'd give you fifty-fifty. But that's just for getting to America and not to do the cycling.'

401

Mike nodded. 'We'll book you in for chemo next week. The nurses will ring you with a day for starting this and we'll scan you in eight weeks' time to see if there have been any changes in your disease.'

'Right. Thank you,' I said and stood pulling on my coat, getting ready to leave.

'Have a good Christmas,' Dr Perrin said.

'You too,' I replied, dropping the soggy tissue in the bin as I left the room.

MIKE

Wearing his best coat and woolly hat, Steven was standing on the path outside my mum's house waiting for me to join him. As I shut the door, he looked up at me, held out his gloved hand expectantly and I took it and we headed off on our short walk to the petrol station to buy a paper. It was a cold December day. Steven's bright blond hair poked out at angles from beneath his hat as he bobbed up and down beside me. He looked the very picture of innocence. My heart constricted knowing what I had to do. It was Jane's idea. She'd thought it best if I explained to him the deterioration in her health 'man to man'.

In the five years since Jane's diagnosis I'd cried only twice – once at renewing our wedding vows in June 2001 and again at a play we'd seen in Adelaide about a boy unable to give his mum a mother's day card. My hat trick came when we heard that Jane's cancer had spread to her liver. We'd always been told that when the cancer moved to any of Jane's visceral organs – her liver, her kidneys, her heart – that it would be a matter of months. I sobbed. Jane watched silently. There was nothing either of us could say to comfort the other.

Steven and I rounded the corner to the petrol station. The lights advertising the garage franchise were dim as a result of the drizzle engulfing the town. The forecourt was empty and the car park behind it the same.

'Steven?'

'Yes, Dad.' He looked up in anticipation.

'You know mum is going to die,' I said.

'Yes, Dad,' he said and I looked down at him as our walk became no more than a shuffle.

'Well, Mum's just had some more scans and the cancer has spread to her liver.' He looked up impassively. 'It means that Mum may not have too much time left with us.'

'Oh.' His voice trembled.

'The doctor said that normally someone as ill as mum might live one year, sometimes two, but sometimes less.'

Steven looked me in the eye. 'Does it depend on how well she reacts to treatment, Dad?'

'Yes. So the most important thing is to make the most of the time we have.' I crouched down to ensure our faces were at the same level. A tear was forming in his eye. His face was twitching, struggling to hold it back. 'It's okay, Steven, it's not soft to cry.'

I leant forward and took him into my arms and hugged him. His arms reached around my neck and he began to sob. Five years ago at the last time of abject desolation he was three and had no concept of how it would affect his life. I waited, allowing him to purge the sadness from his system before saying, 'When we get back, let's not show Mum we're sad though.'

'Okay, Dad,' he said, nodding his head and pulling back from me. I wiped his eyes and playfully hit his chest.

'Oi!' he said, flinging a right hook, knocking me temporarily off balance. 'Are we still going to America?'

'I wouldn't have thought so.'

I decided to take some time off work and spend Christmas at home with the family. The bank has been exceptionally good at providing me sufficient flexibility to be with Jane when needed. Because of the seriousness of Jane's condition, the combination of chemo and Herceptin started in the break between Christmas and New Year. We were both relieved that she would be fitted into the schedule sooner rather than later as psychologically it felt better to be doing something positive rather than leaving the tumour going untreated.

While Jane's mum accompanied her for the treatment, Steven and I stayed at home and played. An IV room is no place for an eight-year-old, so we filled our day playing with the bigger toys which would get under people's feet when the house was busy. I was surprised to get a call from Jane at one o'clock, I'd presumed she wanted me to go to collect her.

'Mike, I've had a reaction to the treatment.'

'Are you all right now?'

'Better than I was,' she said. I detected a slight tremor in her tone, which I found quite worrying. 'But they've stopped giving me my treatment; I need to see Dr Perrin this afternoon.'

'Oh.'

'What do you want to do?' she asked.

'I'll get someone to look after Steven,' I said. 'I'll come over to the hospital.'

It was a slow drive to St James's as sales shoppers were blocking the roads into towns in the late Christmas rush hour. Before I'd even got into the clinic, I ran into one of the IV nurses in the corridor.

'Jane caused quite a stir this morning,' she said. 'We've not had a reaction like that for a while and never with Herceptin.'

'Is she all right?' I asked.

'Yes, she was shaken up for a while though.'

I went through a blue door and Jane was in the seat furthest away, a blanket draped over her lap. 'Dr Perrin's got my notes,' she said, indicating we wouldn't have a long wait.

'Are you okay?'

'Yes,' she said. 'But they just couldn't give me any more Herceptin.'

'How much did you have?'

'Hardly any, it was almost instantaneous.'

I had an irrational loathing of Herceptin. The papers hailed it as a breast cancer wonder drug and there were hundreds of emotive stories of women convinced that without it they'd got a death sentence. But it had almost certainly caused Jane heart damage. She'd been taking it for quite a

405

while until it was discovered, just before 'Rome to Home', that her heart was damaged. Initially there were some doubts over the results because with the amount of damage Jane had, it was felt she'd struggle to walk upstairs. The test was repeated two further times with the same results before it was accepted as genuine. No one had explained in the interim how someone with such a poor function test could complete an ironman. I'd always wondered why the drug manufacturer had not contacted us to do some research into how Jane managed in the circumstances. There seemed to be a whole host of questions, none of which were being answered. It provided no comfort to us when Jane was planning further events that at any point her heart could fail.

'What about the chemo?' I asked.

'I've not had any.'

I had pinned my hopes on starting to attack the tumour today, as we'd no time to lose. Jane could sense my anxiety. 'What?' she asked.

'When will you have some?'

'I don't know.' I fiddled nervously with my hands. 'I know you are worried, it's all over your face, but it's not helping.'

'I'm not.' I tried to sit back in my chair and look as nonchalant as possible, hoping that I could fool her. But it was no use.

'What are they going to do if you can't have the Herceptin, will they give you the chemo?'

Jane's face deflated like a balloon expelling air. 'Look, Mike, I'm as worried as you are. It looks like we're running out of options.

CHAPTER 12

June 2006

MIKE

Although we had all travelled to New York together, I had flown ahead to San Francisco with Michael from the charity SPARKS and Steven, while Jane stayed in New York to do some US media.

She arrived late the following afternoon. As she came into the living room of the house we'd rented, it was instantly noticeable to everyone that she had a pronounced limp on her left side.

She smiled, but then her face dropped as she noticed the bike box which had been wrecked thanks to the cack-handed care of the aircraft baggage handlers. 'Oh,' she said flatly, running her hands along the battered cardboard casing.

'It's good to see you.' I rose from my chair. 'How was your journey?'

'I'm a bit sore.'

'Hi, Jane, how're you doing?' Michael greeted Jane. He was here to help us with the first two weeks of the ride. 'Can I help with your bags?'

Ryan followed Jane in a few seconds later. 'Hello, sirs,' he said cheerily. 'It's good to see you.'

I acknowledged Ryan with a smile, but was too

busy watching Jane as she hobbled round the bike box to take a closer look. Watching her struggling to move, I knew that we were asking too much of her to start the ride. She looked like she couldn't even cycle to the corner shop, let alone over 3000 miles across the United States of America.

'Is there any damage done?' asked Ryan, pointing to the bike box.

'The wheel's buckled, but I'm not sure if any of the kit has gone,' I said.

By eight o'clock, within only a couple of hours of them arriving, Ryan was asleep, Steven tucked in and Michael, Jane and I were in the living room. Jane collected some cushions from other chairs and placed them around her, grimacing as she did so.

'Are you all right?' I asked.

'No. My bum is so sore I can't sit down and I feel dreadful.' She continued to fidget before standing up. With her left arm, she started to massage her lower back, then tried once again to get comfortable in her seat. 'I don't think I'll be able to start the ride if I feel like this. I don't even know if I can sit on a bike.' She started to cry, deep sobs breaking forth. 'Oh, I'm so sore.'

When I stood to go over and comfort her, she waved me away. 'I can't do this,' she said.

'It doesn't matter.' I hovered near her, unsure whether or not to hug her. 'We can just catch a plane home at the weekend. At least we got here – no one would have bet on that at Christmas.'

Jane sat weeping, inconsolable, a lost, frail figure propped up by a multitude of cushions.

'Mike's right, Jane. No one expects you to do this,' said Michael.

She was still crying. 'Jane,' I said. 'You are not well. Everyone understands that and if they don't they can fuck off. The only person that matters is you. Nothing else is important.'

'Exactly,' Michael added.

'But *I* expect me to do this,' said Jane, lifting her head up to look at us both. Her eyes were red-rimmed, streaks of water glistened on her cheeks. She struggled to talk between sobs. 'I have to set off. Sky and ITV have spent thousands of pounds on satellite trucks. Look at all Leeds Metropolitan University have done to help us, Ryan, Martyn, everyone. I'll be letting them down. And think of all those people who will criticise me.'

'Forget Sky and ITV,' I said. 'No one will blame you – they know how poorly you are. Let me call Becca and her friend and tell them not to fly out Friday. We can get a plane home at the weekend and be back at work on Monday. Either way, though, we need to make a decision of some sort tonight.'

Jane was silent. 'Let's go home,' I said quietly. 'That's what we agreed if this situation arose.'

I looked across at Michael, his brow crinkled with concern. After a few moments, Jane took a deep breath and tried to compose herself. 'I don't know what to do,' she said. 'I feel desperately ill. I don't know if I can sit on a bike let alone ride one.'

We sat in silence for five minutes before she said, 'I don't have any choice really – I have to start at least; everyone's spent so much money getting us to this point.'

'No, Jane, let's go home,' I insisted.

She shook her head. 'Let Becca and Jodie travel out Friday. I'll see if I can sit on the bike tomorrow. If I can manage I'll do the pre-day Thursday. If I'm poorly on Friday, I'll not cycle. Give it a couple of days to see if things improve; if not we'll go home.' Jane looked across and forced a smile through the pain. 'I don't want any cameras in my face as I try the bike tomorrow, though.'

'No problem,' I said.

'I mean it, Mike.'

Mid-afternoon the next day, Jane rode her bike for 600 yards. 'How was it?' I asked when she returned.

'I can't tell. Sore.' She was struggling to lift her leg over the frame. I didn't say anything. 'I'll do as we discussed last night.'

After a pleasant reception held in Jane's honour at the British Consulate General's house in San Francisco, we ate out and were back at the accommodation by eight. Jane hobbled across the bedroom, using her arms to prop herself against the bed so as to take the strain off her legs.

'I'm going to take some morphine to try to get on top of the pain so I can rest tonight.'

'What!' I said. We had always agreed that if Jane's condition was so bad that she had to use morphine, she wouldn't do the event. We'd always said that was the line we wouldn't cross.

Jane looked at me, defiance in her eyes. 'I just need to get on top of these spasms in my back and I'll be fine. Just one night to give me a chance to start.' It wasn't an appropriate moment to start a row, so I let the moment pass.

Only twelve hours later we were assembled beneath the Golden Gate Bridge. For once the mist wasn't shrouding its towering red frame which stretched out into the distance.

Jane looked a little edgy, fretting over the bike, her gloves, the timings of the press interviews. Yet I was sure I could detect a little extra spring in her step. Steven was standing with my mum and a family friend, Kathy, who'd travelled up from Los Angeles. I watched him as he stood filming with a hand-held camera and I smiled.

The suspension bridge was a breathtaking sight and I stood admiring the astonishing feat of engineering. It was a beautiful structure – strong and solid yet the ropes gave it a certain fragility. I looked at Jane and we caught each other's eye for a second. There was almost no hope of her completing this ride – we both knew that. Today's skirt through the city was simply an exercise for the media – tomorrow would be the first full day of the event.

Within a minute she was away. Slowly the wheels turned, as she stood on the pedals gently testing her body, almost refusing to take her position on the saddle in fear of the discomfort that would follow. Within seconds, she was about a hundred metres down the road. Only 672,000 to go.

JANE

Pulling on the still unfamiliar cycling gear,

including the white top with the Jane's Appeal and other logos across the front, I hoped that my legs and back would hold out for the first proper stage of cycling.

We were driving around the bay in San Francisco instead of taking the ferry because I couldn't risk the boat ride upsetting my balance at the beginning of the trip. Michael from the charity SPARKS was supporting us on our mammoth journey across America. Ryan sat next to me dressed in the same outfit as mine, holding his cycling helmet in his hands. Our bikes were in the back of the hire car. There was silence in our vehicle. It was too early for conversation. I had not slept well; the nerves about what lay ahead stopped my mind from relaxing.

We arrived at the ferry terminal to find that Martyn, who was filming our adventure en route, had just arrived. His feet clicked on the road as the metal cleats from his cycling shoes hit the surface. He lifted his road bike from the boot of the car and wheeled it round to join ours. Three black bikes with 'Jane's Appeal' standing out in white lettering on the frame. The bikes were all the same, although mine was slightly smaller.

'I can't believe we're here,' I said. Ryan laughed. 'Of course we're here and we're going to be in New York in two months' time.' His voice echoed around the empty parking lot. He bent over the bike and sprayed lubricant on the chain. 'We're good to go, guys.'

Peering at my map, I clicked the detail on the small GPS unit attached to my bike. 'Straight down this hill to the end and turn left.'

Michael was looking at us through the viewfinder of his camera. 'I'll pick up the RV and go on to book somewhere for tonight. I'll ring you later. Be safe.' Rob from *Sky News*, who had come to watch us setting off, wished us well. We all turned and waved one last time and then wheeled the bikes on to the road.

The two men mounted their bikes with ease. I struggled; my back solid and unmoving against the pain, my legs unbending. Finally I managed to throw my leg over the crossbar and push my bottom on to the saddle. 'Right, let's go.' The traffic lights swung from the cable strung across the road. Just one small detail that told us we were in America not Britain. They turned to green and we set off, turning once more to wave at Michael and Rob.

We set off up the broad road rising to the next set of lights and the next. After a gradual climb to the edge of Vallejo, we would be on the road towards Rockville. The rest of America seemed to stretch before us. Large trucks pushed by, their wheels higher than us, the turbulence they created making me wobble on my bike. 'Get off the road,' shouted one truck driver who slowed down to yell at us, 'before you get killed!' He sped off, the gravel spitting from his rear wheels clanking against the fibreglass helmet on my head.

'Charming,' I thought and carried on circling my legs, riding to the right of the white line on the hard shoulder of the road through the debris created by the traffic.

We passed the quarry where the trucks were

headed, the road emptying so that for a while we could ride three abreast, stretched across the road. We cycled for miles along the traffic-free lane next to a busy highway and I watched as the two fitter men quickly crested each hill. I plodded onwards and upwards, my legs grinding round and round to the top of each one until I could swoop downhill again.

'It's really pretty. I thought it might be much more industrial,' Martyn observed. In fact, once we had left the quarry behind, the roads had indeed grown quiet and the lanes narrowed. We had left the city behind us and moved into farmland. We carried on through Rockville and Fairfield until we saw a sign: Winters 10 miles. This was where we were due to meet Michael in one of the RVs. Our first day of cycling was almost over and we could look forward to our first night sleeping in the RVs – motorhomes – that were going to provide our accommodation for the trip.

Four days into the ride and we had a challenging day ahead of us. Michael had dropped us off at the fire station at a small town called Rescue. The temperature had soared to 120 degrees Fahrenheit the day before and a combination of lack of fluids and standing too long in the sun had made Martyn suffer the first signs of heatstroke. He'd slowed himself right down for the last part of the ride and taken all the measures to prevent it getting any worse. But it was good to see him looking less gaunt than when we had finished the afternoon before.

We cycled away from our supporters down the valley to the start of a mammoth 8,500-foot mountain. Carson Pass would take us over the Sierra Nevada range of mountains and into the deserts and salt plains at the other side.

'We need to make sure we keep hydrated,' Ryan said. 'Drink every two miles or every ten minutes, that should be enough.' I nodded and took a long drink from my water bottle. The first hills behind us, we climbed slowly. Using my smallest gear, I watched as Ryan climbed the slopes with ease. We carried on climbing, each rise followed by a very small descent and then another rise. Along Pleasant Valley we gained a lot of height and paused as a small town came into view. I looked at my map: this would be the last town for another thirty miles. We stopped there to fill our water bottles, our last chance for quite a while.

I looked at my watch. It was only nine thirty in the morning, but we still had over forty miles to go, all of it uphill. We crested each hill and glided a small way down before climbing up and up. We'd left the last house behind an hour ago although it seemed that we were not alone. In the woods on the hillside, I could hear the thunder of guns cracking in quick succession. It was a public holiday and people were out hunting and enjoying themselves. At times it sounded as if they were moving closer to us. I pedalled harder to try and keep up with Martyn and Ryan, but found it difficult to reach them and so ended up just a few yards behind, too far to shout up to them to wait. Another clatter of guns and I cycled on. Looking up, I could see Ryan and Martyn stood astride their bikes, waiting for me.

The climb started to get harder; the small downhill slopes disappeared. The sun rose in the sky and the temperature crept up. The road wound its way from the bottom of the valley round and round up this green-clad mountain. The trees shaded us from the full heat but, as I neared another bend, I groaned. I knew that once we turned we would be climbing up the next slope in the full glare of the sun. Martyn's face dropped as he stared ahead of us. I forced the bike on, sweat dripping down my face and arms. Pulling my sunglasses from my face, I wiped the drips from my brow, pushed my glasses back on and kept going. Sweat gathered across my forehead again and slid down my face into my stinging eyes.

I reached a small area of shade and clicked the button on my GPS unit to check our altitude. My heart sank when I saw we had climbed only 4000 feet. We had the same effort to make all over again before we reached the top. I climbed from the bike and sat down in the shade to rest myself.

'How're you doing?' Ryan drawled.

'I'm shattered. I don't think I can do the same again. We've still got so much climbing ahead of us.' As I spoke, tears rose in my eyes and my shoulders hunched round my chest as a sob escaped from my mouth. 'I just don't know if I can carry on up here.'

Martyn sat quietly by the roadside. 'You're doing really well. It's a hard day and it's gonna be tough, but we'll get there. Let's have a few minutes' rest and get going again. We'll see how far we can get.'

I rose after several minutes with a resolve to get

to the top and started moving once more up the slope. The sun beat down. I ground the pedals round until the top of the slope was reached and turned the corner to face the next. Making it to the top of each rise was a victory: a small height gained, a tiny slope nearer the top. My heart sank each time we turned and faced the climbs in the full sunlight. They were the hardest. I would aim for the smallest shadow, the tiniest bit of relief from the heat, and stand there panting, regaining my breath. I crawled up each slope, cycling sometimes only yards before my legs ached too much to go any further.

At last we reached the final slope. We would climb the peak at Carson Pass the following day, but now we had reached our highest point of the day's journey. We had only to coast down towards Silver Lake to finish.

The last mile swooping down the slopes was sweet. Arriving at our destination, I couldn't believe I'd got through the day. My legs were trembling with the effort of the long hours on the bike and I sat heavily on the bench, my head hanging low, waiting to be collected and thinking of the thousands of miles we still had left to go.

'Good cycling, Jane,' said Ryan.

'I'm glad it's over with and we're here. Thanks for your help. I really couldn't have managed otherwise.'

MIKE

I was desperate to get more miles under our belts.

417

Jane's journey over Carson Pass had been tense because the means of communication was so poor. San Francisco was soon left behind and the road to Reno completed as the sun's rays were reflecting off the highway. Trying to concentrate, I caught the latter part of an announcement on a local radio station advising that the road between Reno and Carson City was closed to RVs.

Dismissing it as a trick of hearing, I continued through Reno only to see a large flashing motorway sign warning all RVs and campervans to pull off. Knowing I was only ten miles from Jane, I ignored it. Within seconds the RV was being slung from side to side by winds whipped up off the plain. I gripped the wheel, mouthed a prayer and counted the miles on the milometer.

It was a stark introduction to American climatic extremes, but meeting up with Jane was worth it. She looked well and there was a sparkle in her eye that I hadn't seen over the past year.

The following morning I rose early to see the three riders depart on their way to Fallon. It marked the beginning of their ride across the Nevada and Utah deserts. Within minutes of their departure, Rebecca, Jodie, Steven and I drove to the strip mall for supplies. Infuriatingly, it was impossible to walk between stores without clambering over walls or dodging traffic on the roads. Conscious that we'd been instructed to interview locals for the programme that was being made by Radio Five Live, I entered Starbucks and searched for suitable candidates. As we were about to traverse the desert on Highway 50 – 'America's Loneliest Highway' – I hoped someone could paint a picture of it. The responses from the customers contained the same refrain: 'We don't go on Fifty'. It was as if there was a magnetic field protecting the road. As there were only three routes out of town, I struggled to comprehend how people could live there for decades without using it.

Today was Independence Day and in the evening Fallon was set to celebrate. It was a small town of 8000 people, but the biggest we'd see for 250 miles until we reached Ely. The revelry consisted of 'dirt racing at Rattlesnake Stadium' with fireworks. With Jane feeling unwell, we decided to remain in the RV park. The following morning, we set off across the Salt Wells Basin.

The Salt plain was beautiful, flat and ours. A naturally formed sand mountain offered majesty and recreation. The route navigated its way through a ribbed plain and the climbs came every twenty miles. The telegraph poles were the only indication of human intervention on the landscape. A sign at Middlegate gave the population as eighteen with the number crossed out and replaced by seventeen. Jane wasn't made to feel welcome. It was a male-dominated town so she quickly remounted to ride on to Cold Springs.

There was no need for a population marker at Cold Springs. With one wooden building marked 'Bar Café Gas', it looked like an outpost from the Wild West. Hearing warnings from the bartender to watch out for rattlesnakes, none of us felt particularly comfortable. Cold Springs was in stark contrast to San Francisco, but its solitude, iso-

419

lation and the sense that nature was enveloping you was some experience.

'Did you see the crickets?' Jane asked as she pulled into Austin, Nevada, the next day.

'What crickets?'

'Are you joking? They were hideous, like a plague of locusts across the road. You must have seen them. The stench of the dead ones was like rotting fish; I nearly gipped.'

'Mike, you must have,' Ryan joined in.

'There were thousands.' Jane shook her head and walked off. Rebecca brought over some cutlery and started setting up the wooden table which was between the RVs and the Baptist church. The camp was blessed with minimal facilities, but it was sufficient and cheap. During the late afternoon a collection of locals had driven up, looked at the vehicles, then driven off, which unnerved us all slightly. So when a red pick-up pulled up and a thickset man got out wearing a black T-shirt, we looked at each other nervously.

'What you all doing here?' His voice boomed with more than a hint of menace as he took a few steps towards us.

'We're just staying here tonight,' Michael said.

'We're cycling across the country to raise money for Cancer Research,' Ryan added.

'I heard as much. I'm Bill, the preacher of this church, and I welcome you into our community of Austin. How you liking it?' I eyed up his T-shirt which I'd presumed was advertising a satanic heavy metal band but now noticed it read, 'The

Lord's work'.

'Do you always have so many crickets?' Jane asked.

'Funny you should say that. Until three years ago we didn't have any, then the last two years there've been millions, all over the main street, climbing over our houses. They cause a terrible mess eating everything. It's just between here and Eureka. Last year they caused six fatalities on the roads. Only last night a local man overturned his car on the road up there.' He pointed above his head to the road that snaked up. 'He's seriously hurt. The crickets walk across the road, get run over and make the roads slicker than oil.'

'How do you get rid of them?' Jane asked, looking quite disgusted.

'With a snowplough and then we have to sand down the road.'

'Let's be careful out there tomorrow,' I said. 'We'll take the two RVs through at the same time very slowly.'

It was all we needed.

JANE

'It can't be done,' said Howard, the owner of a small café in Escalante. 'I've been cycling all my life and there's no way physically possible that you can cycle from Escalante River all the way to Hanksville in one day.'

'Well, that's what we're going to do and that's where we're hoping to finish tomorrow,' I said. 'We'll just have to see how far we can get.'

'It's too hard a day, and too harsh out there for you to go ninety-six miles.' Howard opened his arms wide to emphasise his point. He handed Ryan his card. 'If you do by any chance make it – and you won't – give me a phone call on this number. I'd love to hear from you.'

Ryan took the card. 'We'll ring you tomorrow night then.' He looked at me.

I shrugged my shoulders. 'Maybe it'll be too far. We'll just have to see how it goes.'

We headed back to the small RV park at the edge of the town. 'See you at five thirty for breakfast then,' Ryan said. I scrunched my face up in disgust at the thought of rising from bed so early yet again.

The next morning we drove through the canyon we had cycled down the day before. The view was spectacular from the top, layer after layer of mesa, the flat-top mountains typical of the area. Yesterday the white-and-gold-striated mountains had glowed orange under the full glare of the afternoon sun. Now, the early morning light made them a creamier colour. Mike hit the brakes and passed slowly down the same steep gradient we had screeched down on bikes yesterday at speeds in excess of 40 m.p.h. I had sped down not daring to touch on my brakes, trusting I would make it round the corners, then surprised by the clatter of the cattle grid under my wheels at the very bottom of the slope.

We rounded the last bend to find a parking area. I climbed into the living quarters of the RV and picked up my cycling helmet which contained the last few things I needed. I placed my phone and inner tube in the pockets at the back of my cycling shirt, along with an energy bar and some power gels to replace the sugars I would be using up as I struggled with the heat and the climbs later on in the day.

At the start of each day there were the small preparations, pumping up the tyres, lubricating the chain, checking the brakes, filling water bottles and attaching our panniers. This morning our reluctance to start on such a long day meant we'd prevaricated over these last-minute tweaks until Ryan called us to the task in hand. Martyn and I followed him to the road and we started the long climb up towards Boulder Town.

Even this early in the day the heat was building up. The sun hadn't penetrated the more sheltered canyons, but the radiance from the day before had been stored in their striped walls and the heat built up in the low valleys, making us stop within a couple of miles to take off some of our layers of clothing.

I stood astride the bike and breathed in before continuing, the dry heat making my breath harsh. Finally we crawled to the top of the ridge where large volcanic rocks were in evidence, dark brown and porous-looking, strewn across the landscape. Then we were cycling across the Hogsback, a ridge with sheer drops to either side. The day was calm, the wind light. Otherwise we would have felt extremely precarious on the narrow lanes that lead towards Boulder Town.

We met the RVs at Boulder Town and sat in the air-conditioned haven for a few moments. Filling our water bottles, drinking sweet iced coffee and munching on frosted pastries restored some of the energy we had used over the last couple of hours' exertions. Ready for the road again, we set off after only twenty minutes, having arranged to meet Mike once we'd got over the 9000 foot peak at Homestead Overlook. The sun high up in the sky, sweat already glistening on our arms and legs, we set off.

It was eleven miles to the top of the climb. But it was a slow eleven miles. The heat meant that we had to stop every two miles to seek some shade. At last we were on the final reach up to the top. As I looked behind me, two cyclists were gradually gaining on us up the hill, their blue and red T-shirts a familiar sight. On several occasions over the last couple of weeks they had passed us, but we hadn't exchanged words, just acknowledged each other with a nod and a lift of the hand. They passed us as we crested the top and stopped at the familiar large RVs.

Mike was there, Steven beside him, his face obscured by his small video camera.

'What was that like, Mum?' he asked.

'Hot and hard,' I told him, 'a really tough climb.'

Our next stop was Torrey. My back ached and there was a hollow pit of hunger in my stomach which I tried to fill with a sandwich and a sweet iced coffee. The two cyclists who had passed us earlier were refuelling at the same sandwich shop. They looked gaunt, the haunted look in their eyes the first stages of dehydration. They looked how I felt.

'We're over halfway through today's ride,' Ryan said. 'Let's push on through the next set of canyons and see how we feel.'

The day was hard, the heat savage, the roads full of potholes. I felt as if my tyres were sticking to the road, each mile requiring a huge effort. I sat heavily on the saddle, the tiredness in my legs and back making me hunch my shoulders and clutch tightly at the taped handlebars. We moved from an open landscape to a more sheltered valley. The walls of the canyon created a local wind tunnel effect, so that the hills that had previously been tortuous suddenly seemed less steep. I flew along between the tall red walls, my speed pushing from 12 m.p.h. to over 20 m.p.h. Suddenly the miles were speeding by, and on my GPS I could see the distance we still had to cover falling by huge jumps. I hung my head down low over the handlebars and turned my legs, lifting the drink bottle from its cradle to take a drink, then replacing it, every ten minutes. I lowered myself as the miles sped by and started to feel lighter on the bike. The tiredness of earlier in the day had gone.

We were cycling close to a small river which helped to cool the road. On a small stretch of grass I saw two familiar bikes laid down, the panniers removed, their young riders nowhere in evidence. I knew they must be bathing in the river and part of me wanted to leave my bike by the roadside and do the same, savour the cool flowing water in such an arid land. I looked at my watch, the day was passing and if I didn't continue there was no way we could make it the remaining miles to Hanksville. The cool canyon had helped claw back some precious mileage and time which I couldn't waste.

I'd caught glimpses of Ryan and Martyn round each turn ahead of me. We had pushed on each at our own pace, aware of one another but cycling alone. Close enough to call out if we had problems, far enough away to keep our own speed. The miles kept clicking down until we reached Caineville, the last stop of the day before our final destination of Hanksville.

'So what do you think?' I asked Ryan and Martyn. 'Do we carry on or stop here?'

'It's up to you,' they replied in unison.

'I feel okay. I know I'm well hydrated and I'm confident that I can cycle another eighteen miles. Shall we go for it?'

We climbed upwards, the road curling between two canyons striped yellow, cream and red. At the top a new and even more barren landscape was laid out before us. Gone was the palate of colour; everything before us was grey and dusty.

'It could be the scene of the lunar landing,' said Martyn. Small craters were in evidence like ulcers on the landscape. There were small rises in the distance across the otherwise flat plain. We carried on towards Hanksville, willing ourselves on the last ten, then nine, then eight miles until we saw a small green oasis in the distance.

It took us another ten minutes to reach the one-lane town and our weary bodies welcomed the sight of the two RVs. I collapsed on a bench.

'So are you going to ring this bloke then?' Ryan asked.

'Here, I'll ring him.' Mike punched in the numbers. Howard was stunned at the news that we'd done the journey to Hanksville in one day. "You lot are awesome," he says, "unbelievable",' Mike reported as he finished the call.

We were glad of the day before's decision to push on when we set off at 6 a.m. the following day. I was looking forward to wading through the cool fresh waters of the Colorado River in the evening. The heat in Utah continued unabated. Temperatures soared up and reached over 110 degrees Fahrenheit. The next two days' cycling felt as if we were pushing ourselves and our bikes through a roaring hot oven.

'What are we doing to ourselves?' Martyn asked as we drank yet another bottle of tepid water to slake our thirst. Each mile was an enormous effort.

'I feel like a kebab skewered on my bicycle saddle,' I said as we pushed on along the heat-ridden road, the canyon ahead of us distorted by the heat haze, the road a silvery slick of unreal water.

I didn't get to cool my toes in the Colorado River. The bridge took us hundreds of feet above it and even if we could reach it, the year's drought had made it just a mere muddy trickle. At the other side of the dried-up Lake Powell, we had the climbs of Colorado to look forward to. We could just make out the bluish outline of the Rockies; the huge challenge to come.

MIKE

Jane looked as nervous as if she were hovering at the edge of an open aeroplane door. The altitude certainly matched that of many parachute jumps. She fretted with her helmet strap.

We'd been at altitude for a number of days and Jane had suffered nosebleeds, nausea, lack of appetite and breathlessness. Her weight loss was visible to all and her eyes were receding back into her skull. 'You'll be all right,' I tried to reassure her.

'I know, I just want to get on with it.' Monarch Pass at 11,312 feet was the high point of the ride and the final big climb in the Rockies.

'Are we ready?' Jane shouted across the forecourt of the café where we had stopped. It was a twelve-mile climb of 3000 feet. Jane was conscious of the risks; any weakness of her heart would be ascertained in the next ninety minutes. She put her foot on the pedal and was off. We agreed to meet them every three miles on the ascent, partly to provide drinks, but it would also reassure me that she was fine.

After two stops at the three- and six-mile point, I waited three miles from the summit as Ryan came towards me. 'She doesn't want to stop.'

'How is she?' I asked.

'Bloody fantastic, sir. She's eating up the road.' I knew that was unlikely as I'd been up all night with her, her back causing her incredible pain. I'd gently massaged it through the small hours, but

428

it was the morphine once again which dulled the pain. The danger of someone breaking the guidelines once is that they will continue to do so and now morphine was the regular treatment when Jane had taken all the Co-proxamol she was allowed.

Jane drew alongside me, her mouth open wide, gulping in as much air as she could. Her fingerless black gloves gingerly gripped the handlebars. I sensed the lack of sensation in them was causing distress. Her cheeks were sinking in like an old man taking part in a gurning competition. Over the last few days the ride had changed from an adventure to survival. 'Are you okay?' I asked.

There was no reply as she took another lungful of air, her helmeted head nodding in time with the rotation of the pedals. Martyn followed her, his cheeks flushed. Monotonously, Jane continued her rhythmic cadence as first a huge lorry and then our RV passed. At the top we didn't have long to wait before Martyn, then Jane and Ryan arrived. I sighed with relief as Jane approached. After photos, phone calls and a dodgy hot dog, we contemplated what to do next. Should we descend straight away or ride the small cable car to the mountain summit 800 feet higher?

'Let's do the cable car, Mike, I haven't done anything touristy on the ride.' Jane knew my fear of heights. 'Don't be soft.' Reluctantly I agreed and the eight of us made our way into two cars. It was our first cool day and now the clouds began to look threatening. Although it was only a ten-minute journey I began to feel a little panicky. Fortunately I faced forward so couldn't see the huge drop behind me.

'I could jump from here,' I said to no one in particular in an attempt to reassure myself. Then there was a tap on the roof as if someone wanted to come in, quickly followed by two or three more.

'Hailstones,' said Jane, as the marble-sized objects rattled. It felt as if we were trapped inside a steel drum. A lightning bolt lit up the ever-darkening sky. 'Don't worry.' I felt the colour draining from my face.

Within a couple of minutes the elderly ride steward was unlocking the door and I clambered out quickly, following Steven but ahead of Jane.

'I've had to shut the ride down during the storm,' he said. I noticed that the cable was still. 'There are three floors including this one; the next one is an enclosed observational tower and above that an open tower. Please don't go on to the top floor or outside as it's dangerous because you are at a summit. This floor is earthed, but you'll be safer on the second.'

The lightning was beginning to break out in various locations. I put my arm on Steven's shoulder. 'What about the car behind us?'

'What car?' the steward asked.

'The car with the other four people in our party.'

'I didn't know there was anybody else.' He pressed a button and the equipment sprung into life, the cable started to slowly move around and, within a couple of minutes, Rebecca, Jodie, Martyn and Ryan appeared. We were on the highest point for miles and the storm was breaking out all around; lightning lit up the sky every couple of seconds.

'How often do you get storms round here?' I asked.

'Every few days but only one a month like this. It'll be over in a minute.' From the darkness of the sky and the amount of lightning strikes, which seemed to be closing in, that seemed unlikely. A bolt crashed near us and the steward quickly put his radio to his ear.

'The shop's taken a direct hit. It's blown out every lightbulb in the building, glass everywhere.' Suddenly sparks lit up the outside of the tower, followed by an almighty crack as the observation tower took a direct hit. The steward involuntarily jumped back a couple of feet.

He regained his composure. 'Don't worry; we're perfectly safe. I jump easily.'

Steven held on to Jane. 'I'm scared, Mum. I don't want to go down on the cable car.'

'It's okay. We won't be doing anything until this storm has passed. I'm glad we didn't set off cycling.'

I looked out of the window and the road was completely white from the hailstones. Further down, the crews had temporarily stopped cleaning up the wreckage of yesterday's car crash in a similar hailstorm. Again there was a massive crack and sparks crackled from the exterior of the building, which coincided with the steward taking an involuntarily leap six feet backwards. His attempt to reassure us carried little weight this time.

On each side the skies were illuminated by fierce lightning bolts. Steven hugged his mum and for the first time Jodie and Rebecca edged back in their seats. Within thirty minutes the storm had passed. The cable car was inoperable because the lightning had frayed the cables, so the owner of the ride drove us down the mountain peak.

'I've lived here all my life,' he said, 'and that's the worst storm we've had.' Perhaps Jane was safer in the saddle after all.

JANE

The last days in Colorado had been so flat we felt as if we were already cycling through Kansas.

'Look, there's a bend in the road up ahead.' Ryan was squinting from behind his sunglasses into the distance.

Following his gaze, I could see a small rise in the road, which did indeed bend to the right. 'That's at least three miles away,' I said.

'No, one mile at the most,' Ryan replied. 'What do you reckon, Martyn?'

'Oh, I'd say about two.' We continued cycling and it was about eight minutes later when we finally arrived at the slight twist in the road. 'Just over two miles,' I said. 'Well, that was exciting! What next to look forward to?'

The road was long and straight. On our left was a railway line with telegraph poles following its course. Something strange had happened to the poles and they seemed to be shorter and shorter as we went along, until the lines they held aloft barely cleared the ground. On our right was an endless field of corn. The height of the corn gave

432

us a small amount of protection from the diagonal cross-wind that we'd been forcing our way through all morning. It wasn't a strong wind, but the continual pressure made our progress seem much slower than it actually was. The huge distances between the tiny urban areas took an age to cover. We could see water towers held aloft on their grey stilted legs from as far away as twelve miles. Reaching them was our target but they never seemed to get any nearer.

A bare metal pole came into view. 'Look,' said Ryan, 'somebody's stolen the Kansas sign.'

'What?' I replied, pulling myself from the hypnotic state of cycling.

'This is the state border. We've entered the fifth state of our ride.'

'Oh good. One state nearer home.'

'Don't be like that, Jane,' said Martyn. 'I'm really enjoying the landscape. It's much more interesting than I thought it would be.'

I laughed. 'You're kidding, right?'

'No. It's just fantastic to be here.'

The cycling became more difficult as the sun grew hotter. It seemed that the heat whipped the wind up from the road, the hot air impeding our efforts even further. Still we drew up at Tribune, our end point for the day, just after midday, relieved to have covered the fifty-eight miles in about four and a half hours.

'What took you?' Mike asked as we dismounted from our bikes.

'Well, that's a great way to greet us,' I responded.

'I'm only joking.' His face lit up with a grin.

'Recovery drinks all round?'

The high protein and carbohydrate drinks had been a godsend. They allowed me to replenish lost nutrients even when we were cycling through the high altitudes in Colorado and nausea had overtaken me and made it almost impossible to eat. We opened the cans and upended them, drinking the sweet contents quickly. Then we gulped down water to wet our dry parched throats.

The sun was high that afternoon when we went to explore the local town, the heat only made bearable by the wind that blew us along the street. We passed boarded-up shops and a bowling alley that must have been long closed. There was Tina's Cut 'n' Curl still doing business and a small chemist. Everybody else seemed to have left town. At the main crossroads a single traffic light hung from the cables, the orange light showing in all directions. The wind picked up and sent it swinging alarmingly over the road, the cable squeaking and creaking.

'Where's that music coming from?' Mike asked.

'Up there, Daddy,' said Steven, his brown cowboy hat pushed low on his head. 'Hotel California' was playing mournfully from four speakers at each corner of the crossroads. We stood watching this eerie scene, not another soul in sight. The town seemed abandoned, the spell only broken when a black Chevy rolled up to the junction, stopped and then rolled on down the road. The driver gave the slightest of waves, acknowledging us as we passed.

The wind that had blown us up the main street

made us put our heads down as we struggled back to the town's only motel and our sleeping quarters for the night.

'I hope the wind drops, otherwise it's going to be hard work cycling tomorrow,' I said.

'And hard work driving this thing.' Mike's hands extended in an open gesture around the RV. 'It acts like a sail and the wind really pushes you around when you're driving along the road.'

'You'll be fine. We'll set out early again so you'll be off the road by ten and we'll be finished by one-ish.'

I stared out of the window the next morning before I pulled on my cycling gear. It seemed a little calmer than the night before. Once on the bike, though, the wind kept pushing the bike and me three feet across the road. It took all my concentration to stay on and not allow the front wheel to slide away from me. As the heat increased, so did the wind. I was glad to see the sign for Dighton, our end point for the day.

I started singing a mantra to myself as each mile went by, 'Seven more miles to go, seven more miles to go' to the tune of 'One Man and His Dog'. At last we passed into the city limits and I was relieved to think I could finish our day's cycling. I stepped off the bike and unclipped my helmet, glad to be safe at the end of another day.

MIKE

The bedclothes rustled. A foot gently touched

435

the floor, a second later an 'Ow' as the foot collided with a bag.

'Bloody, bloody RV.' Jane stumbled and lurched to the toilet door. I felt her side of the bed which appeared to have had half a dozen buckets of water thrown over it. Each night she had been sweating profusely, regardless of the air temperature.

'How are you?' I asked when she returned.

'My back's bad.'

'Do you want me to rub it? What's the time?' Jane climbed back on to the bed. By her body outline I could tell she was moving with considerable difficulty.

'It's four. I'm not quite sure what to do with myself.'

'I'll rub your back.'

'I'm too sore to sit up. Can I lie down?' I moved my fingers gently across her back, trying not to apply too much pressure. 'Not on the bone or side ... be careful,' she muttered.

'Sorry.'

'No, I'm sorry for being so pathetic.' She wasn't. I couldn't imagine the pain she was going through. My hand was barely touching her skin, yet it was as if my fingers were charged with static electricity.

After thirty minutes she said, 'You can stop now, get some sleep. There's no point in both of us being tired.'

I continued gently stroking the painful area before Jane eventually stopped me. 'Will you pass me the morphine?'

I sighed quietly. This had been a regular feature

of most nights or early evenings, Jane relying on morphine to supplement her other painkillers. I readjusted my position and grabbed the box containing the bottle. 'You know we agreed–'

Jane stopped me. 'You don't need to remind me, but I'm in so much pain that there is no alternative if I want to be able to get on the bike.'

'We could just go home. You don't have to put yourself through this torture. It's not as if we are raising any money at the moment. It's all pointless. Let's get up, pack the RV and shoot off to the airport. We could get a flight from Indianapolis today; we'd be home by tomorrow and start making you feel comfortable.'

Jane sat up and emptied two plastic spoonfuls of morphine into her mouth. 'I have to finish for us to get the charities enough money to make the ride worthwhile. It's only by finishing that we'll raise any money, you know that.'

'Jane, you're too ill. No one should have to go through this amount of pain. It's inhumane.'

Jane slumped back down on the bed, her hair matted, her pyjamas so wet that they were likely to give an impromptu shower. 'I have to finish, we've gone so far and there's no money yet.' She started to cry out in desperation and pain.

'Whatever you want to do, but I think we should go home.'

Jane sobbed quietly.

Half an hour later, at five o'clock, she was climbing out of bed to begin the preparations for the morning's ride. Outside it was at least one hour until dawn, the sounds of any wildlife drowned out by the generator on our sister RV as

Ryan prepared his morning bagel. Jane clunked clumsily around the bed. There was so little space that our bags were left strewn on the floor at night. As she had so little movement in the morning, each day started with her tripping up. She pulled on her cycling top, her torso now so skinny that the tight-fitting lycra hung loose. I hadn't seen her so thin for years and she looked terribly unwell.

'Did you sleep okay?' Jane asked.

'Did you?' Neither of us needed to answer.

Steven was asleep in his bed above the driver's cab. He, too, was beginning to look tired as the journey took its toll. 'What have you decided to do?' I asked Jane, although I knew I was looking at the answer as she stood before me in full cycling kit.

'I'm going to set off. The morphine has eased the pain and now I can take some Co-proxamol. The spasms have gone out of my back so at least I can move about a little. What time are you seeing us?'

'We'll be at the first stop. I can't persuade you to come to the airport then?' There was no response and within seconds the RV door rattled shut.

JANE

We set off from Pine Grove just inside the north-western border of West Virginia, down the valley road, following the path of the river. A single train track meandered towards and away from the road as it rose and dropped with the vale. I approached each tight corner with trepidation. I shook my head to listen out for the warning growls and barks of any guard-dogs that might have heard us.

A continuous yapping sent Ryan ahead. He turned and raised his thumb. 'It's okay!' he yelled. 'They're in a pen.' I carried on, pushing the pedals round, forcing the bike forwards. The sound of the barking grew in intensity and ferocity as two large black dogs hurled themselves against the metal grid of their small pen. Letting out a sigh of relief, I continued after Ryan as he headed onwards.

I dropped into the smallest ring and clicked through the gears until I reached one I felt I could use to climb the small incline steadily, but would still be able to stand up on the pedals and sprint away from any impeding attacks.

My chest was tight, my ribs ached from the last four days of similar climbs. Slow, searching cycling followed by sprinting away from dogs baring their teeth, snarling and yapping, tails down, eyes wide as they threw themselves from the hillside properties when they heard the creaking of our bikes.

Another hill, another tight corner at the top of it. The quiet of the valley was broken by the sound of the hounds' baying close at hand. It echoed through the hillside and was caught up by other dogs. I pushed myself hard and sprinted over the peak of the hill towards the relief of a downhill, keeping the houses in sight as dog after dog, black and brown hunting hounds, hurled themselves towards us. My chest expanded. Unable to let my breath out, my ribs resisted the tightness and screamed with pain.

'Jane, it's okay. They're chained,' Ryan was calling out. Each dog snapped to a halt as the furthest extent of its chain was reached, then they stood on hind legs baying at us, eyes gleaming as they tested their restraints. I freewheeled to the bottom of the hill and stopped my bike. I let out my breath. I was dizzy with the strong adrenalin rush, dizzy from holding my breath with fear.

I dismounted and hung my head, shielding my face with my hands as the weeks of coping with my phobia of dogs finally overcame me. 'Oh shit. Oh shit. Oh shit.' I spoke softly into the palms of my hands trying to shut out the world. 'Oh shit. Oh shit. Oh shit.' I started to rock back and forth to feel some comfort, to take away the deep scared feeling that tightened my stomach and my throat, clamping my lips together.

'What is it, Jane?' Martyn asked in alarm as I sat, a broken woman, sobbing by the roadside miles from anywhere. I shook my head, not trusting myself to talk just yet.

'Jane, it's okay. The dogs are chained. It's fine.'

'What if they hadn't been?' I said finally. 'How could I have got away from them? There were so many.'

'Ryan and I would have been there. They wouldn't have got near you.'

'I'm just so scared and I don't want to feel like this any more. I don't want to get up in the morning and be scared for the next sixty miles of cycling. It's making me feel so ill. I just don't think I want to do this to myself any more. It's not worth it.'

'Come on,' Martyn urged. 'Think of New York. It's not so far now.'

'That's just it. We've been cycling like this for weeks, and I've been telling myself it'll be all right, it'll be worth it when we get to New York. Now I've just stopped caring whether we get there or not.'

Martyn moved to one side to give me time to calm myself and Ryan pulled up alongside. 'Is everything all right?' He looked at me and drew away to speak in a quiet voice with Martyn. I sat enveloped by my own fear, unable to bring any clarity to my situation. I couldn't face another mile of cycling if there was a chance I might meet with even one more dog.

Ryan returned. 'Listen, Jane. You don't have to carry on if you don't want. It's up to you. Take all the time you need. We'll just sit here.'

'I know. Thank you. It's not rational this fear, but I can't help it.'

'Martyn and I won't let a dog near you. You have my word on that. There's no way they'll get past us.' I smiled weakly at Ryan. A small calm voice inside me was trying to talk to my quivering, fearful self until I was confident enough to push myself up from my resting place.

'Right then.' I sighed deeply. 'I suppose we'd better get on. Otherwise the others will be wondering where we've got to. And it'll be a very long day.' The two men grinned at me and we cycled on through the green clad valley.

MIKE

'Your shoelaces are undone,' I told Jane as she climbed into the lift of the Staten Island Hotel.

'I know.' She'd saved a new pristine-white cycling top for the last morning's ride. Her hands were full carrying a bag, two Gatorade bottles and her GPS unit.

'Do you want me to tie them for you?'

'I can manage. My back's very sore and I can't bend down for the first thirty minutes of the day.' It was another reminder of the personal price she'd paid to cross America. For the past four weeks it had become a battle of survival for Jane, tempered by the beautiful views that were so abundant here. The lift came and we descended. My heart sank with the lift. Don't let your paranoia rub off on Steven, I told myself firmly.

'Good luck, Mum.' Jane bent down to Steven and gave him a hug, wincing as she stood back upright. I smiled at the thought that there are some things that will increase the pain threshold. Steven and I, loaded with suitcases, continued on our journey to the car, which we were meticulously packing.

An hour later we'd arrived at Battery Park where Jane was due to finish the ride. We had planned to have a celebration that night at Mr Kays in New York, where we had eaten after the New York Marathon last year. But Jane was now so unwell that we were going to take the first available flight home so we could try to make her comfortable as soon as possible. In the circumstances we'd also decided to have a low-key finish. Some New York police officers and cycling clubs had offered to give an escort into Manhattan and the finish, but Jane is never one to have a fuss made of her.

In truth, we hadn't decided where the finish would be, but left it up to Rob to decide when the *Sky News* crew arrived that morning. It had been a long few months since we'd been told that Jane's cancer had spread to her liver and I don't think any of us believed this moment would happen. Only two days earlier Jane had looked beaten, but like a prizefighter dragging himself from the canvas in the fifteenth round, she had risen and continued. To all of us who had seen her it was obvious that she was incredibly unwell; gaunt, hobbling, her left arm almost permanently resting on her back.

As the minutes ticked by until Jane, Ryan and Martyn approached Battery Park, I saw the crowd of media people grow, together with some visitors from Yorkshire. Putting my hand on Steven's shoulder, I steered him away from everyone into an oasis of calm a few yards away. I sunk to my knees.

'I love you, Steven.'

'I love you too, Dad.'

'Remember this moment for the rest of your life as your mum finishes the ride. Realise you can achieve the impossible and you won't go far wrong in life. Mum's here and alive because of you, Rebecca and Suzanne. No one else, just you three.'

'And you, Dad,' said Steven.

443

AFTERWORD

On 1 September 2006, six years after being told she had only six months to live, Jane finished her nine-week, 3700-mile Ride Across America from San Francisco to New York. She lost a quarter of her bodyweight in the process. It was hailed as one of the greatest endurance feats ever undertaken by a terminal cancer sufferer. Her husband, Mike, called it 'a celebration of human spirit over the body's frailty' and said he had seen Jane dig deeper than ever before.

At the time of going to press, the Tomlinsons have raised over £1,425,000 for charity.

ACKNOWLEDGEMENTS

The journey is no easier now than in 2000 but without the ongoing support of family and friends it would be substantially more difficult. During these adventures there have been a small but dedicated group of people who have given invaluable assistance: Luke and his family Karen, Sue, Peter and Tom; Ryan Bowd and Martyn Hollingworth.

Our employers, the National Australia Bank and Leeds Hospital Trust, have continued to provide consistent invaluable support without which most of these events wouldn't have taken place. You don't raise the vast sums of money we have without the support of companies, the media and most importantly the individual members of the public who have made un-solicited donations in their tens of thousands.

Our charity will continue to help those children and cancer patients most in need and you can find details of how you can assist on www.janesappeal.com.

It only leaves us to thank those who have helped on the book: Jill Foster again for her patience, Joanne for having to put up with our tapes, Mark Lucas at LAW and all the team at Simon & Schuster.

The publishers hope that this book has given you enjoyable reading. Large Print Books are especially designed to be as easy to see and hold as possible. If you wish a complete list of our books please ask at your local library or write directly to:

Magna Large Print Books
Magna House, Long Preston,
Skipton, North Yorkshire.
BD23 4ND

This Large Print Book for the partially sighted, who cannot read normal print, is published under the auspices of

THE ULVERSCROFT FOUNDATION

THE ULVERSCROFT FOUNDATION

... we hope that you have enjoyed this Large Print Book. Please think for a moment about those people who have worse eyesight problems than you ... and are unable to even read or enjoy Large Print, without great difficulty.

You can help them by sending a donation, large or small to:

**The Ulverscroft Foundation,
1, The Green, Bradgate Road,
Anstey, Leicestershire, LE7 7FU,
England.**
or request a copy of our brochure for more details.

The Foundation will use all your help to assist those people who are handicapped by various sight problems and need special attention.

Thank you very much for your help.